PHARMACOLO
CALCULATIONS
FOR NURSES:

A WORKTEXT

Third Edition

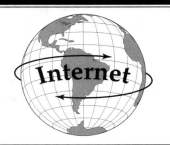

PHARMACOLOGICAL CALCULATIONS FOR NURSES:

A WORKTEXT

Third Edition

PEGGY H. BATASTINI,
R.N., C., M.Ed., M.S.N.

Director of Associate Degree Nursing Program
Associate Professor of Nursing
Columbus State University, Columbus, Georgia

JUDY K. DAVIDSON,
R.N., C.S., B.S.N., M.N.

Associate Professor of Nursing
Columbus State University, Columbus, Georgia

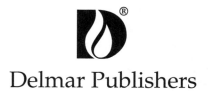

Delmar Publishers

an International Thomson Publishing company I(T)P®

Albany • Bonn • Boston • Cincinnati • Detroit • London • Madrid
Melbourne • Mexico City • New York • Pacific Grove • Paris • San Francisco
Singapore • Tokyo • Toronto • Washington

NOTICE TO THE READER

Cover Design: Carol D. Keohane

Delmar Staff
Publisher: William Brottmiller
Acquisitions Editor: Marion Waldman
Production Coordinator: Barbara A. Bullock
Project Editor: Patricia Gillivan
Art and Design Coordinator: Jay Purcell
Editorial Assistant: Diane Speece

COPYRIGHT © 1999
Delmar is a division of Thomson Learning. The Thomson Learning logo is a registered trademark used herein under license.

Printed in the United States of America
    5 6 7 8 9 10 XXX 03 02

For more information, contact Delmar, Learning, Executive Woods, 5 Maxwell Drive, Clifton Park, NY 12065; or find us on the World Wide Web at http://www.delmar.com

International Division List

Japan:
Thomson Learning
Palaceside Building 5F
1-1-1 Hitotsubashi, Chiyoda-ku
Tokyo 100 0003 Japan
Tel: 813 5218 6544
Fax: 813 5218 6551

Australia/New Zealand
Nelson/Thomson Learning
102 Dodds Street
South Melbourne, Victoria 3205
Australia
Tel: 61 39 685 4111
Fax: 61 39 685 4199

UK/Europe/Middle East:
Thomson Learning
Berkshire House
168-173 High Holborn
London
WC1V 7AA United Kingdom
Tel: 44 171 497 1422
Fax: 44 171 497 1426

Latin America:
Thomson Learning
Seneca, 53
Colonia Polanco
11560 Mexico D.F. Mexico
Tel: 525-281-2906
Fax: 525-281-2656

Canada:
Nelson/Thomson Learning
1120 Birchmount Road
Scarborough, Ontario
Canada M1K 5G4
Tel: 416-752-9100
Fax: 416-752-8102

Asia:
Thomson Learning
60 Albert Street, #15-01
Albert Complex
Singapore 189969
Tel: 65 336 6411
Fax: 65 336 7411

Library of Congress Cataloging-in-Publication Data

Batastini, Peggy H.
        Pharmacological calculations for nurses : a worktext / Peggy H.
    Batastini, Judy K. Davidson.—3rd ed.
            p.   cm.
        Includes index.
        ISBN 0-7668-0166-7
        1. Pharmaceutical arithmetic. 2. Nursing. I. Davidson, Judy K.
    II. Title.
        [DNLM: 1. Pharmaceutical Preparations—administration & dosage
    nurses' instruction. 2. Pharmaceutical Preparations—administration
    & dosage programmed instruction. 3. Mathematics nurses'
    instruction. 4. Mathematics programmed instruction. QV 18.2 B328p
    1999]
    RS57.B36   1999
    513'.024'615—dc21
    DNLM/DLC   98-46290
    for Library of Congress   CIP

Contents

Preface

Accurate calculation of drug problems can be explained simply and clearly. We have found, however, that many textbooks on the market utilize complicated formats, multiple methods of problem solving, and unnecessary material that must be clarified and/or omitted.

We based this textbook on the assumption that learners want to know methods that will enable them to solve drug problems with simplicity, ease, and accuracy. In each chapter we provide basic rules and formulas, example problems, and multiple practice problems. Each learner is the best judge of how many practice problems are necessary to master nursing math skills.

In this third edition, the authors responded to suggestions from nursing students, faculty, and reviewers—and included additional information in several areas of the text. Unit objectives are identified. Key terms are bold where first defined for clarity. Answers to practice problems are placed at the end of each chapter. A new chapter explains the "How To's" of medication administration, including: How to use Universal time, how to read a drug label, how to understand medication schedules, and understanding common abbreviations. Outdated medications are deleted, and a substantial number of new practice problems are added. The entire section on titrated drugs is revised to reflect current nursing practice. Drug labels are incorporated into parenteral practice problems.

This worktext is designed to be used as a self-teaching text or to be used within an organized course. We believe that clear explanations, multiple practice problems, and comprehensive tests will help the learner gain confidence and accuracy in solving drug problems.

Peggy H. Batastini
Judy K. Davidson

Columbus State University
Columbus, Georgia

Acknowledgments

Reviewers

Carol Boswell, RN, EdD
Chairman, Department of Nursing
Odessa College
Odessa, Texas

Dorcas C. Fitzgerald, MSN, RN
Associate Professor of Nursing
Youngstown State University
Youngstown, Ohio

Elaine Ridgeway, RN, MSN
Assistant Professor of Nursing
Clayton College and State University
Morrow, Georgia

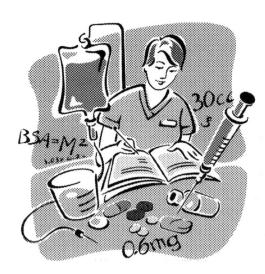

UNIT 1

Arithmetic Skills Review

Unit Objectives

Upon completion of this material, the learner will be able to:

- Add, subtract, multiply, and divide fractions and decimals.
- Reduce fractions to lowest terms.
- Change percentages to numerical and decimal fractions.
- Change numerical and decimal fractions to percentages.
- Set up and solve ratio and proportion problems.
- Express simple numbers in Roman numerals.

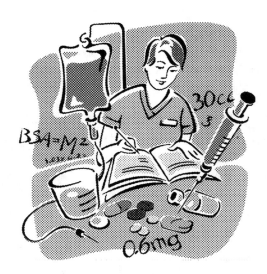

CHAPTER 1

Numerical Fractions

In mathematical problems for nurses, we use **whole numbers** and fractions. A **fraction** represents a part or portion of a whole number. If a pie is divided into six equal pieces, each piece is $\frac{1}{6}$ of the pie, as seen in Figure 1.1.

One-sixth ($\frac{1}{6}$) is a numerical fraction. The **numerator** is 1 and the **denominator** is 6.

FIGURE 1.1

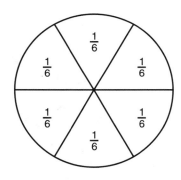

The line between 1 and 6 means divide.

The fraction $\frac{1}{6}$ can be read one-sixth, or one divided by six.

Terms	
$\dfrac{1}{6}$ ← Numerator ← Denominator	
$\dfrac{7}{6}$	Improper fraction
$1\dfrac{1}{6}$	Mixed Number

Reducing to Lowest Terms

The numerator and the denominator are the **terms** of a fraction. Consider the fraction $\frac{30}{80}$. We wish to reduce the size of the numbers without changing their value.

RULE

> You can multiply both terms of a fraction by the same number, or divide both terms of a fraction by the same number, without changing the value of the fraction.

EXAMPLE: Knowing that rule, look again at $\frac{30}{80}$. We want a number that will divide evenly into both terms. In this case, 10 will divide into both terms.

$$30 \div 10 = 3 \qquad 80 \div 10 = 8$$
$$\frac{30}{80} = \frac{3}{8}$$

Furthermore, there is no number that will divide evenly into both 3 and 8, so the fraction $\frac{3}{8}$ is said to be in **lowest terms**. Lowest terms are the simplest terms of a fraction.

EXAMPLE: Reduce to lowest terms: $\frac{16}{20}$.

With your knowledge of multiplication tables, you see that *4* will divide evenly into both *16* and *20*.

$$16 \div 4 = 4 \qquad 20 \div 4 = 5$$
$$\frac{16}{20} = \frac{4}{5}$$

STEPS

To reduce a fraction to its lowest terms:

1. Determine the largest number that divides evenly into both numbers.
2. When the fraction cannot be reduced any farther, it is in its lowest terms.

PRACTICE PROBLEMS—REDUCING TO LOWEST TERMS

Reduce to lowest terms:

1. $\frac{10}{12}$ 3. $\frac{16}{32}$ 5. $\frac{38}{70}$ 7. $\frac{3}{9}$

2. $\frac{20}{48}$ 4. $\frac{100}{150}$ 6. $\frac{6}{24}$ 8. $\frac{3}{18}$

9. $\frac{10}{25}$ 12. $\frac{75}{150}$ 15. $\frac{12}{108}$ 18. $\frac{40}{100}$

10. $\frac{44}{124}$ 13. $\frac{15}{60}$ 16. $\frac{5}{35}$ 19. $\frac{50}{1000}$

11. $\frac{60}{180}$ 14. $\frac{32}{64}$ 17. $\frac{25}{225}$ 20. $\frac{18}{117}$

Changing an Improper Fraction to a Mixed Number

STEPS

1. Divide the denominator into the numerator. (This gives the whole number.)
2. Write the remainder over the denominator. (This gives the fraction.)

EXAMPLE: Change $\frac{16}{5}$ to a mixed number.

$$\text{Denominator} \longrightarrow 5\overline{)16} \longleftarrow \text{Numerator}$$
$$\underline{15}$$
$$1 \longleftarrow \text{Remainder} \quad \frac{16}{5} = 3\frac{1}{5}$$

REMEMBER

A **mixed number** is lowest terms of an improper fraction.

PRACTICE PROBLEMS—CHANGING AN IMPROPER FRACTION TO A MIXED NUMBER

Change the following improper fractions to mixed numbers and reduce them to lowest terms:

1. $\frac{11}{7}$ 5. $\frac{13}{6}$ 9. $\frac{39}{2}$ 13. $\frac{250}{30}$

2. $\frac{16}{3}$ 6. $\frac{35}{9}$ 10. $\frac{110}{15}$ 14. $\frac{61}{7}$

3. $\frac{27}{8}$ 7. $\frac{127}{11}$ 11. $\frac{44}{3}$

4. $\frac{5}{4}$ 8. $\frac{54}{5}$ 12. $\frac{69}{6}$

Changing a Mixed Number to an Improper Fraction

STEPS

1. Multiply (×) the denominator by the whole number, and then add in the numerator.

2. Place that number over the denominator.

EXAMPLE: Change $1\frac{7}{8}$ to an improper fraction.

$$8 \times 1 = 8 \qquad\qquad 8 + 7 = 15$$
$$1\frac{7}{8} = \frac{15}{8}$$

PRACTICE PROBLEMS—CHANGING A MIXED NUMBER TO AN IMPROPER FRACTION

Change the following mixed numbers to improper fractions:

1. $3\frac{3}{4}$ 5. $9\frac{10}{11}$ 9. $12\frac{1}{6}$ 13. $16\frac{1}{8}$

2. $2\frac{1}{2}$ 6. $6\frac{2}{3}$ 10. $4\frac{11}{15}$ 14. $6\frac{4}{5}$

3. $5\frac{7}{8}$ 7. $20\frac{7}{10}$ 11. $10\frac{7}{9}$

4. $1\frac{1}{5}$ 8. $8\frac{1}{4}$ 12. $11\frac{1}{3}$

Finding a Common Denominator

When fractions have the same denominator, we say they have a **common denominator**. We cannot add or subtract fractions with unlike denominators.

STEPS

To discover a common denominator, find a number into which both denominators will divide evenly. Often, you can do this by knowing the multiplication tables. If a number does not easily come to mind, simply multiply all the denominators together, and that will give you a common denominator.

EXAMPLE: Find the common denominator for these two fractions: $\frac{5}{11}$ and $\frac{4}{13}$. Multiply the denominators to get a common denominator of 143.

$$11 \times 13 = 143$$

Next, divide the denominator of each fraction into the common denominator 143.

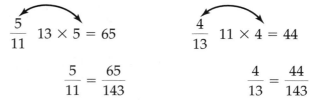

$$\frac{5}{11} \quad 143 \div 11 = 13 \qquad\qquad \frac{4}{13} \quad 143 \div 13 = 11$$

Quotient   **Quotient**

Next, take that quotient and multiply it by the numerator of each fraction.

$$\frac{5}{11} \quad 13 \times 5 = 65 \qquad\qquad \frac{4}{13} \quad 11 \times 4 = 44$$

$$\frac{5}{11} = \frac{65}{143} \qquad\qquad \frac{4}{13} = \frac{44}{143}$$

EXAMPLE: Find a common denominator for $\frac{3}{8}$ and $\frac{5}{6}$. From the multiplication tables, we know that both *8* and *6* will divide evenly into *24*. Furthermore, we know that *24* is the *smallest* number into which *8* and *6* will divide evenly. Twenty-four is termed the *lowest* common denominator.

To change $\frac{3}{8}$ and $\frac{5}{6}$ to fractions with the denominator 24:

$$\frac{3}{8} \quad 24 \div 8 = 3 \qquad\qquad \frac{5}{6} \quad 24 \div 6 = 4$$

$$3 \times 3 = 9 \qquad\qquad 5 \times 4 = 20$$

$$\frac{3}{8} = \frac{9}{24} \qquad\qquad \frac{5}{6} = \frac{20}{24}$$

PRACTICE PROBLEMS—FINDING A COMMON DENOMINATOR

Find the lowest common denominator for the following fractions:

1. $\frac{1}{2}$ and $\frac{1}{3}$ 4. $\frac{1}{5}$ and $\frac{3}{4}$ 7. $\frac{2}{3}$ and $\frac{2}{4}$

2. $\frac{2}{3}$ and $\frac{2}{5}$ 5. $\frac{1}{4}$ and $\frac{5}{8}$ 8. $\frac{11}{12}$ and $\frac{2}{5}$

3. $\frac{1}{2}$ and $\frac{3}{8}$ 6. $\frac{4}{5}$ and $\frac{1}{2}$ 9. $\frac{15}{16}$ and $\frac{3}{4}$

10. $\frac{3}{7}$ and $\frac{1}{2}$ 16. $\frac{1}{5}$ and $\frac{3}{6}$ 22. $\frac{15}{48}$ and $\frac{16}{25}$

11. $\frac{2}{7}$ and $\frac{1}{3}$ 17. $\frac{7}{12}$ and $\frac{16}{21}$ 23. $\frac{5}{8}$ and $\frac{4}{5}$ and $\frac{2}{4}$

12. $\frac{4}{5}$ and $\frac{5}{9}$ 18. $\frac{10}{13}$ and $\frac{15}{25}$ 24. $\frac{3}{8}$ and $\frac{5}{7}$ and $\frac{8}{9}$

13. $\frac{4}{8}$ and $\frac{11}{9}$ 19. $\frac{25}{50}$ and $\frac{20}{60}$ 25. $\frac{2}{10}$ and $\frac{5}{6}$ and $\frac{1}{8}$

14. $\frac{6}{12}$ and $\frac{2}{11}$ 20. $\frac{10}{100}$ and $\frac{30}{36}$

15. $\frac{14}{16}$ and $\frac{1}{8}$ 21. $\frac{3}{10}$ and $\frac{5}{7}$

Addition of Fractions

STEPS

1. Find a common denominator.

2. Add the numerators together and write over the common denominator.

3. Reduce to lowest terms.

EXAMPLE: Add $\frac{1}{6}$ and $\frac{4}{12}$. The common denominator is 12.

$$\frac{1}{6} = \frac{2}{12}$$

$$\begin{array}{r} \frac{2}{12} \\ + \frac{4}{12} \\ \hline \frac{6}{12} = \frac{1}{2} \end{array}$$

$\frac{6}{12}$ reduced to lowest terms is $\frac{1}{2}$.

Addition of Mixed Numbers

STEPS

1. Write the mixed numbers in a column.

2. Add the fractions; reduce to lowest terms.

3. Add the sum of the fractions to the sum of the whole numbers.

EXAMPLE: Add $3\frac{7}{8}$ and $2\frac{3}{8}$.

$$3\frac{7}{8}$$
$$+\,2\frac{3}{8}$$
$$\overline{5\frac{10}{8}}$$

Change $\frac{10}{8}$ to a mixed number.

$$\frac{10}{8} = 1\frac{1}{4}$$

Add $1\frac{1}{4}$ to $5 = 6\frac{1}{4}$.

$$5\frac{10}{8} = 6\frac{1}{4}$$

PRACTICE PROBLEMS—ADDITION OF FRACTIONS

Add the following fractions and reduce them to lowest terms:

1. $\frac{4}{6}$ $+\frac{3}{8}$

2. $\frac{5}{9}$ $+\frac{2}{3}$

3. $\frac{6}{8}$ $+\frac{1}{4}$

4. $\frac{2}{3}$ $+\frac{5}{4}$

5. $\frac{3}{4}$ $+1\frac{3}{5}$

6. $\frac{7}{9}$ $+\frac{5}{6}$

7. $\frac{3}{10}$ $+\frac{2}{5}$

8. $\frac{3}{8}$ $+\frac{7}{12}$

9. $\frac{2}{3}$ $+\frac{5}{7}$

10. $\frac{5}{9}$ $+\frac{4}{3}$

11. $\frac{5}{8}$ $+\frac{2}{6}$

12. $\frac{1}{2}$ $+\frac{3}{5}$

13. $\frac{4}{9}$ $+\frac{1}{2}$

14. $\frac{5}{15}$ $+\frac{3}{10}$

15. $\frac{6}{8}$ $+\frac{2}{16}$

16. $5\frac{2}{3}$ $+7\frac{3}{5}$

17. $4\frac{7}{8}$ $+12\frac{7}{24}$

18. $6\frac{3}{5}$ $+1\frac{3}{4}$

19. $3\frac{7}{10}$ $+9\frac{4}{15}$

20. $16\frac{1}{8}$ $+4\frac{3}{10}$

21. In the hospital gift shop, a patient bought $\frac{3}{4}$ lb of caramels, $\frac{2}{3}$ lb of chocolate, and $1\frac{1}{2}$ lb of peanut brittle. How many pounds of candy did she buy?

22. Mrs. Jones added $\frac{1}{8}$ tsp cinnamon, $\frac{1}{16}$ tsp cloves, $\frac{3}{4}$ tsp nutmeg, and $1\frac{1}{4}$ tsp vanilla to a batch of cookies. How much spice did she use?

23. Mrs. Thomas gave birth to twins. One baby weighed $2\frac{3}{4}$ lb, and the other weighed $3\frac{3}{5}$ lb. What was the combined weight of the babies?

24. If Mrs. Brown freezes $2\frac{3}{8}$ lb of blackberries, $9\frac{2}{10}$ lb of peaches, $6\frac{3}{5}$ lb of cherries, and $5\frac{1}{4}$ lb of strawberries, how much fruit will she freeze?

25. In a coffee shop, Jane bought $\frac{1}{3}$ lb of one type of coffee and $\frac{6}{15}$ lb of another. How much coffee does Jane have?

Subtraction of Fractions

STEPS

1. Find a common denominator.
2. Subtract the numerators; write the answer over the common denominator.
3. Reduce to lowest terms.

EXAMPLE: Subtract $\frac{2}{12}$ from $\frac{4}{12}$.

$$\begin{array}{r} \frac{4}{12} \\ - \frac{2}{12} \\ \hline \frac{2}{12} \end{array}$$ ($\frac{1}{6}$ in lowest terms)

Subtraction of Mixed Numbers

STEPS

1. Write the mixed numbers in a column.
2. Subtract the fractions; borrow from the whole number if necessary.
3. Subtract the whole numbers.

EXAMPLE: Subtract: $10\frac{1}{5} - 6\frac{3}{5}$.

$10\frac{1}{5}$ ← **To subtract $\frac{3}{5}$ from $\frac{1}{5}$, it is necessary to borrow 1**

$- 6\frac{3}{5}$ **from the 10. One is also $\frac{5}{5}$. Add the $\frac{5}{5}$ to $\frac{1}{5}$.**

The problem is now:

$$9\frac{6}{5}$$
$$- 6\frac{3}{5}$$
$$\overline{3\frac{3}{5}}$$

PRACTICE PROBLEMS—SUBTRACTION OF FRACTIONS

Subtract the following fractions and reduce them to lowest terms:

1. $\frac{4}{3}$
    $-\frac{2}{3}$

6. $\frac{5}{8}$
    $-\frac{7}{12}$

11. $\frac{9}{12}$
     $-\frac{1}{3}$

16. $14\frac{5}{6}$
     $- 12\frac{1}{3}$

2. $\frac{5}{9}$
    $-\frac{1}{6}$

7. $\frac{5}{6}$
    $-\frac{1}{3}$

12. $\frac{18}{21}$
     $-\frac{5}{7}$

17. $13\frac{4}{5}$
     $- 7\frac{1}{10}$

3. $\frac{7}{6}$
    $-\frac{3}{18}$

8. $\frac{7}{15}$
    $-\frac{2}{5}$

13. $\frac{11}{12}$
     $-\frac{5}{16}$

18. $11\frac{12}{15}$
     $- 1\frac{4}{6}$

4. $\frac{13}{20}$
    $-\frac{4}{15}$

9. $\frac{11}{16}$
    $-\frac{1}{4}$

14. $\frac{18}{28}$
     $-\frac{3}{7}$

19. $15\frac{51}{64}$
     $- 2\frac{5}{8}$

5. $\frac{7}{8}$
    $-\frac{2}{3}$

10. $\frac{21}{32}$
     $-\frac{7}{16}$

15. $6\frac{3}{4}$
     $- 2\frac{1}{2}$

20. $15\frac{5}{28}$
     $- 11\frac{1}{7}$

21. A bandage is $5\frac{1}{3}$ ft long. The nurse uses $2\frac{1}{8}$ ft to dress a patient's arm. How much bandage remains?

22. If a woman bought $3\frac{3}{4}$ yd of material and used only $1\frac{1}{5}$ yd for a skirt, how much material would remain?

23. The pharmacy sends $1\frac{1}{2}$ cups of cornstarch for use in a soothing bath. If the patient uses $\frac{1}{3}$ cup, how much cornstarch remains?

24. Mary used $2\frac{1}{16}$ cups flour and $\frac{3}{4}$ cup brown sugar in a batch of cookies. How much more flour did she use than brown sugar?

25. One infant weighs $10\frac{3}{8}$ lb, and another weighs $6\frac{1}{5}$ lb. What is the difference in their weights?

Multiplication of a Fraction by a Fraction

STEPS

1. Multiply the numerators.
2. Multiply the denominators.
3. Write the product of the numerators over the product of the denominators.
4. Reduce to lowest terms.

Terms	
5 ⟵——Multiplicand	
×2 ⟵——Multiplier	
10 ⟵——product	

EXAMPLE: Multiply: $\frac{5}{4} \times \frac{1}{2}$.

$$\frac{5 \times 1}{4 \times 2} = \frac{5}{8}$$

Multiplication of a Fraction by a Mixed Number

STEPS

1. Change the mixed number to an improper fraction.
2. Multiply.

EXAMPLE: Multiply: $7\frac{1}{8} \times \frac{3}{4}$. Change $7\frac{1}{8}$ to $\frac{57}{8}$.

$$\frac{57}{8} \times \frac{3}{4} = \frac{57 \times 3}{8 \times 4} = \frac{171}{32} = 5\frac{11}{32}$$

Multiplication of a Fraction by a Whole Number

STEPS

1. Write the whole number as a numerator, and write 1 as the denominator.
2. Multiply.

EXAMPLE: Multiply: $6 \times \frac{4}{5}$.

$$\frac{6}{1} \times \frac{4}{5} = \frac{6 \times 4}{1 \times 5} = \frac{24}{5} = 4\frac{4}{5}$$

PRACTICE PROBLEMS—MULTIPLICATION OF FRACTIONS

Multiply the following fractions and reduce them to lowest terms:

1. $\frac{3}{4} \times \frac{2}{3}$

8. $\frac{10}{12} \times 32$

15. $1\frac{4}{9} \times \frac{6}{32}$

2. $\frac{1}{3} \times \frac{8}{9}$

9. $\frac{4}{9} \times 10$

16. $4\frac{2}{3} \times \frac{11}{15}$

3. $\frac{7}{16} \times \frac{7}{8}$

10. $\frac{7}{8} \times 15$

17. $5\frac{3}{4} \times \frac{1}{12}$

4. $\frac{3}{5} \times \frac{7}{10}$

11. $\frac{16}{40} \times 5$

18. $11\frac{1}{5} \times \frac{7}{8}$

5. $\frac{5}{18} \times \frac{4}{9}$

12. $\frac{6}{16} \times 17$

19. $15\frac{3}{9} \times 10\frac{2}{5}$

6. $\frac{11}{12} \times \frac{6}{16}$

13. $7\frac{3}{4} \times \frac{1}{2}$

20. $1\frac{16}{31} \times 4\frac{6}{17}$

7. $\frac{5}{6} \times 11$

14. $12\frac{1}{10} \times \frac{2}{5}$

21. $\frac{1}{3}$ of $\frac{1}{2}$ is what?

22. What part of $\frac{2}{10}$ is $\frac{3}{16}$?

23. What part of 15 is $\frac{7}{8}$?

24. A bag of intravenous fluid is infusing at a rate of 61 ml per hour. How much will infuse in $3\frac{1}{2}$ hours?

25. A bottle of medicine contains $16\frac{3}{4}$ oz of liquid. How much liquid is in $7\frac{1}{2}$ bottles?

Division of a Fraction by a Fraction

STEPS

1. Invert the divisor.

2. Multiply the fractions.

3. Reduce to lowest terms.

Terms				
10	÷	2	=	5
↑		↑		↑
Dividend		Divisor		Quotient

EXAMPLE: Divide $\frac{5}{8}$ by $\frac{1}{16}$.

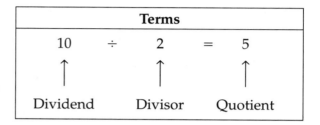

$$\frac{5}{8} \div \frac{1}{16} = \frac{5}{8} \times \frac{16}{1} = \frac{80}{8} = \mathbf{10}$$

Dividend   Divisor   Quotient

REMEMBER

The word *by* stands for the division sign. The number following the division sign is the **divisor**.

Division of a Fraction by a Whole Number

STEPS

1. Write the whole number as a fraction, with a denominator of *1*.

2. Invert the divisor and multiply.

EXAMPLE: Divide $\frac{1}{8}$ by 8.

$$\frac{1}{8} \div \frac{8}{1} =$$

$$\frac{1}{8} \times \frac{1}{8} = \frac{1}{64}$$

EXAMPLE: Divide 4 by $\frac{1}{3}$.

$$4 \div \frac{1}{3} =$$

$$\frac{4}{1} \times \frac{3}{1} = \mathbf{12}$$

Division of a Fraction by a Mixed Number

STEPS

1. Change the mixed number to an improper fraction.
2. Divide.

EXAMPLE: Divide $\frac{7}{10}$ by $1\frac{1}{5}$.

$$\frac{7}{10} \div 1\frac{1}{5} = \frac{7}{10} \div \frac{6}{5} =$$

$$\frac{7}{10} \times \frac{5}{6} = \frac{7 \times 5}{10 \times 6} =$$

$$\frac{35}{60} = \frac{7}{\mathbf{12}}$$

PRACTICE PROBLEMS—DIVISION OF FRACTIONS

Divide the following fractions and reduce them to lowest terms:

1. $\frac{1}{5} \div 4$

2. $\frac{2}{3} \div 6$

3. $\frac{4}{8} \div 7$

4. $\frac{2}{10} \div 5$

5. $\frac{1}{6} \div 7$

6. $\frac{5}{9} \div 8$

7. $\frac{2}{3} \div \frac{3}{8}$

8. $\frac{4}{5} \div \frac{3}{4}$

9. $\frac{1}{2} \div \frac{1}{6}$

10. $\frac{7}{8} \div \frac{5}{2}$

11. $\frac{4}{10} \div \frac{7}{10}$

12. $\frac{5}{8} \div \frac{10}{3}$

13. $\frac{2}{5} \div 1\frac{3}{8}$

14. $\frac{2}{3} \div 1\frac{7}{8}$

15. $\frac{3}{4} \div 2\frac{1}{2}$

16. $\frac{1}{5} \div 5\frac{5}{6}$

17. $\frac{1}{3} \div 2\frac{3}{8}$

18. $2\frac{1}{4} \div 2\frac{1}{3}$

19. $1\frac{3}{10} \div 3\frac{1}{2}$

20. $3\frac{1}{5} \div 1\frac{5}{6}$

21. A can of infant formula concentrate contains $10\frac{3}{4}$ oz, which is enough for four bottles of formula. How much concentrate is needed for one bottle?

22. If a patient receives 569 ml of an intravenous solution in $2\frac{1}{2}$ hours, how much is being administered in one hour?

23. If it takes $133\frac{1}{3}$ yd of cotton fabric to make 50 rolls of bandage, how much fabric does it take for 1 roll?

24. It takes a patient $1\frac{1}{4}$ hours to walk 6 kilometers. How much time does it take him to walk 1 kilometer?

25. A clinic nurse spends $2\frac{1}{2}$ hours interviewing 10 clients. If the nurse spends the same amount of time per client, how long does it take for each interview?

ANSWERS

Reducing to Lowest Terms (pp. 4–5)

1. $\frac{5}{6}$	**6.** $\frac{1}{4}$	**11.** $\frac{1}{3}$	**16.** $\frac{1}{7}$
2. $\frac{5}{12}$	**7.** $\frac{1}{3}$	**12.** $\frac{1}{2}$	**17.** $\frac{1}{9}$
3. $\frac{1}{2}$	**8.** $\frac{1}{6}$	**13.** $\frac{1}{4}$	**18.** $\frac{2}{5}$
4. $\frac{2}{3}$	**9.** $\frac{2}{5}$	**14.** $\frac{1}{2}$	**19.** $\frac{1}{20}$
5. $\frac{19}{35}$	**10.** $\frac{11}{31}$	**15.** $\frac{1}{9}$	**20.** $\frac{2}{13}$

Changing an Improper Fraction to a Mixed Number (p. 5)

1. $1\frac{4}{7}$
2. $5\frac{1}{3}$
3. $3\frac{3}{8}$
4. $1\frac{1}{4}$

5. $2\frac{1}{6}$
6. $3\frac{8}{9}$
7. $11\frac{6}{11}$
8. $10\frac{4}{5}$

9. $19\frac{1}{2}$
10. $7\frac{1}{3}$
11. $14\frac{2}{3}$
12. $11\frac{1}{2}$

13. $8\frac{1}{3}$
14. $8\frac{5}{7}$

Changing a Mixed Number to an Improper Fraction (p. 6)

1. $\frac{15}{4}$
2. $\frac{5}{2}$
3. $\frac{47}{8}$
4. $\frac{6}{5}$

5. $\frac{109}{11}$
6. $\frac{20}{3}$
7. $\frac{207}{10}$
8. $\frac{33}{4}$

9. $\frac{73}{6}$
10. $\frac{71}{15}$
11. $\frac{97}{9}$
12. $\frac{34}{3}$

13. $\frac{129}{8}$
14. $\frac{34}{5}$

Finding a Common Denominator (pp. 7–8)

1. 6
2. 15
3. 8
4. 20
5. 8
6. 10
7. 12

8. 60
9. 16
10. 14
11. 21
12. 45
13. 72
14. 132

15. 16
16. 30
17. 84
18. 325
19. 300
20. 3600
21. 70

22. 1200
23. 40
24. 504
25. 240

Addition of Fractions (pp. 9–10)

1. $1\frac{1}{24}$
2. $1\frac{2}{9}$
3. 1
4. $1\frac{11}{12}$
5. $2\frac{7}{20}$
6. $1\frac{11}{18}$
7. $\frac{7}{10}$

8. $\frac{23}{24}$
9. $1\frac{8}{21}$
10. $1\frac{8}{9}$
11. $\frac{23}{24}$
12. $1\frac{1}{10}$
13. $\frac{17}{18}$
14. $\frac{19}{30}$

15. $\frac{7}{8}$
16. $13\frac{4}{15}$
17. $17\frac{1}{6}$
18. $8\frac{7}{20}$
19. $12\frac{29}{30}$
20. $20\frac{17}{40}$
21. $2\frac{11}{12}$

22. $2\frac{3}{16}$
23. $6\frac{7}{20}$
24. $23\frac{17}{40}$
25. $\frac{11}{15}$

Subtraction of Fractions (pp. 11–12)

1. $\frac{2}{3}$
2. $\frac{7}{18}$
3. 1
4. $\frac{23}{60}$
5. $\frac{5}{24}$
6. $\frac{1}{24}$
7. $\frac{1}{2}$

8. $\frac{1}{15}$
9. $\frac{7}{16}$
10. $\frac{7}{32}$
11. $\frac{5}{12}$
12. $\frac{1}{7}$
13. $\frac{29}{48}$
14. $\frac{3}{14}$

15. $4\frac{1}{4}$
16. $2\frac{1}{2}$
17. $6\frac{7}{10}$
18. $10\frac{2}{15}$
19. $13\frac{11}{64}$
20. $4\frac{1}{28}$
21. $3\frac{5}{24}$

22. $2\frac{11}{20}$
23. $1\frac{1}{6}$
24. $1\frac{5}{16}$
25. $4\frac{7}{40}$

Multiplication of Fractions (p. 13)

1. $\frac{1}{2}$
2. $\frac{8}{27}$
3. $\frac{49}{128}$
4. $\frac{21}{50}$
5. $\frac{10}{81}$
6. $\frac{11}{32}$
7. $9\frac{1}{6}$

8. $26\frac{2}{3}$
9. $4\frac{4}{9}$
10. $13\frac{1}{8}$
11. 2
12. $6\frac{3}{8}$
13. $3\frac{7}{8}$
14. $4\frac{21}{25}$

15. $\frac{13}{48}$
16. $3\frac{19}{45}$
17. $\frac{23}{48}$
18. $9\frac{4}{5}$
19. $159\frac{21}{45}$
20. $6\frac{316}{527}$
21. $\frac{1}{6}$

22. $\frac{3}{80}$
23. $13\frac{1}{8}$
24. $213\frac{1}{2}$
25. $125\frac{5}{8}$

Division of Fractions (pp. 15–16)

1. $\frac{1}{20}$
2. $\frac{1}{9}$
3. $\frac{1}{14}$
4. $\frac{1}{25}$
5. $\frac{1}{42}$
6. $\frac{5}{72}$
7. $1\frac{7}{9}$

8. $1\frac{1}{15}$
9. 3
10. $\frac{7}{20}$
11. $\frac{4}{7}$
12. $\frac{3}{16}$
13. $\frac{16}{55}$
14. $\frac{16}{45}$

15. $\frac{3}{10}$
16. $\frac{6}{175}$
17. $\frac{8}{57}$
18. $\frac{27}{28}$
19. $\frac{13}{35}$
20. $1\frac{41}{55}$
21. $2\frac{11}{16}$

22. $227\frac{3}{5}$
23. $2\frac{2}{3}$
24. $\frac{5}{24}$
25. $\frac{1}{4}$

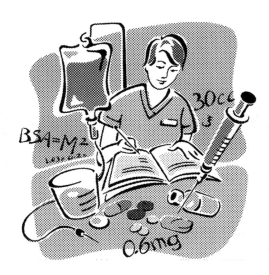

CHAPTER 2

Decimal Fractions

In the world of real numbers, there are whole numbers and fractions of numbers. There also is an imaginary number line that has a point or decimal in the center, as shown in Figure 2.1. Numbers on this line have a *place* value.

FIGURE 2.1

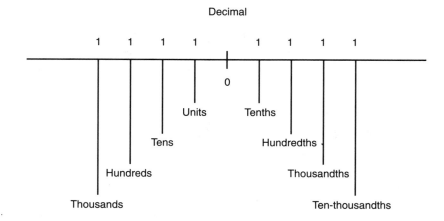

Numbers to the left of the decimal are whole numbers. If no decimal point appears in a number, the decimal is understood to be to the right of the number. The whole number 2 is also *2.0,* with the decimal showing.

Numbers to the right of the decimal are decimal fractions and are read according to their place value:

0.1	one-tenth
0.01	one-hundredth
0.001	one-thousandth
0.0001	one-ten thousandth

REMEMBER

When dealing with decimal fractions (such as one-tenth), always place a zero in front of the decimal—0.1. This prevents one from mistaking the decimal, one-tenth, for the whole number 1.

Addition of Decimal Fractions

STEPS

1. Write the numbers in a column with the decimals aligned.

2. Add as usual, placing the decimal in the answer beneath the decimals in the problem.

EXAMPLE: Add 1.03, 3, 2.146, and 0.02.

$$
\begin{array}{r}
1.03 \\
3 \\
2.146 \\
+\,0.02 \\
\hline
\mathbf{6.196}
\end{array}
$$

PRACTICE PROBLEMS—ADDITION OF DECIMAL FRACTIONS

Add the following decimal fractions:

1.
$$
\begin{array}{r}
19.09 \\
+\,13.47 \\
\hline
\end{array}
$$

4.
$$
\begin{array}{r}
765.13 \\
8.60 \\
13.40 \\
+\;\;52.10 \\
\hline
\end{array}
$$

7.
$$
\begin{array}{r}
0.5 \\
1.4 \\
+\,0.002 \\
\hline
\end{array}
$$

10.
$$
\begin{array}{r}
1.001 \\
0.0005 \\
+\;\;8.2 \\
\hline
\end{array}
$$

2.
$$
\begin{array}{r}
168.39 \\
+\;\;39.19 \\
\hline
\end{array}
$$

5.
$$
\begin{array}{r}
28.30 \\
42.96 \\
+\,132.10 \\
\hline
\end{array}
$$

8.
$$
\begin{array}{r}
3.4592 \\
0.13 \\
+\,52.42 \\
\hline
\end{array}
$$

11.
$$
\begin{array}{r}
10.01 \\
15.0 \\
+\;\;3.2 \\
\hline
\end{array}
$$

3.
$$
\begin{array}{r}
37.40 \\
+\,32.90 \\
\hline
\end{array}
$$

6.
$$
\begin{array}{r}
267.02 \\
529.53 \\
+\,178.35 \\
\hline
\end{array}
$$

9.
$$
\begin{array}{r}
6.89 \\
0.57 \\
+\,22.16 \\
\hline
\end{array}
$$

12.
$$
\begin{array}{r}
0.45 \\
0.29 \\
+\,15.43 \\
\hline
\end{array}
$$

13.   0.73
    39.58
    0.5
    8.7
  + 0.003

15.   5.3
    0.007
    15.2
  + 9.03

17. 140.7
    0.35
    8.047
  + 2.3

19.   40.26
    0.43
    30.49
  + 6.2

14. 125.9
    14.97
    6.66
    0.09
  + 1.1

16.   7.56
    3.5
    28.82
  + 16.25

18.   38.73
    4.9
    6.246
  + 12.8

20.   2.39
    2.68
    5.7
  + 200.013

21. Clinic bill charges are $1.59, $3.58, $0.79, and $0.85. What is the total?

22. Lengths of wood were cut into 15.9-in, 0.5-in, 23.9-in, 17.3-in, and 10-in pieces for a woodworking project. How many total inches of wood were cut?

23. Four patients received hospital bills. The charges were $5,382.00, $13,956.00, $25,005.59, and $18,536.00. What was the total of the four bills?

24. The heights of four boys were measured in centimeters—153.2, 163.18, 175.5, and 179.7. What was the sum of their heights in centimeters?

25. What is the total weight of books weighing 454 g, 579.6 g, 502.01 g, 710.30 g, and 1500.002 g?

Subtraction of Decimal Fractions

STEPS

  1. Write the numbers in a column with the decimals aligned.

  2. Subtract as usual. Place a decimal in the answer beneath the decimals in the problem.

EXAMPLE: Subtract: $16.459 - 0.37$.

$$
\begin{array}{r}
16.459 \\
-\;\,0.37 \\
\hline
\mathbf{16.089}
\end{array}
$$

PRACTICE PROBLEMS—SUBTRACTION OF DECIMAL FRACTIONS

Perform the following subtractions:

1.	$\begin{array}{r}5.8\\-3.7\end{array}$	**8.**	$\begin{array}{r}78.096\\-45.365\end{array}$	**15.**	$\begin{array}{r}13.9929\\-\;\;8.867\end{array}$
2.	$\begin{array}{r}12.3\\-10.09\end{array}$	**9.**	$\begin{array}{r}9.2003\\-7.2183\end{array}$	**16.**	$\begin{array}{r}1.003\\-0.4657\end{array}$
3.	$\begin{array}{r}50.1\\-24.6\end{array}$	**10.**	$\begin{array}{r}12.10001\\-\;\;5.00020\end{array}$	**17.**	$\begin{array}{r}7.604\\-7.60353\end{array}$
4.	$\begin{array}{r}14.06\\-\;\;6.005\end{array}$	**11.**	$\begin{array}{r}26.36902\\-15.29292\end{array}$	**18.**	$\begin{array}{r}30.1\\-19.896\end{array}$
5.	$\begin{array}{r}26.08\\-\;\;9.12\end{array}$	**12.**	$\begin{array}{r}8.3087\\-7.2183\end{array}$	**19.**	$\begin{array}{r}5.132\\-2.9132\end{array}$
6.	$\begin{array}{r}57.34\\-37.49\end{array}$	**13.**	$\begin{array}{r}87.073\\-24.333\end{array}$	**20.**	$\begin{array}{r}3.1\\-0.998\end{array}$
7.	$\begin{array}{r}9.002\\-5.050\end{array}$	**14.**	$\begin{array}{r}111.1\\-\;\;7.001\end{array}$		

21. One patient weighs 57.49 kg, and another weighs 62.15 kg. What is the difference in their weights?

22. Ted's hospitalization cost $15,409.73, and Mike's cost $13,707.95. How much more did Ted pay than Mike?

23. One board is 549.75 cm, and another is 1043.97 cm. What is the difference?

24. Mrs. Jones paid $57.85 for medicine; however, Mrs. Smith's medicines were $105.19. How much more did Mrs. Smith pay?

25. One beaker of water measures 1004.92 ml, and another measures 956.92 ml. What is the difference?

Multiplication of Decimals

STEPS

1. Find the product as usual.

2. Count the number of decimal places in both the multiplicand and the multiplier.

3. Mark off the total number of decimal places in the product and insert a decimal.

EXAMPLE: Multiply: 1.03×0.2.

Step 1:

$$
\begin{array}{r}
1.03 \longleftarrow \textbf{multiplicand} \\
\times \ 0.2 \longleftarrow \textbf{multiplier} \\
\hline
\textbf{Product} \longrightarrow 206
\end{array}
$$

Step 2: Count the number of decimal places in the multiplicand and the multiplier.

$$
\begin{array}{r}
1.03 \\
\times \\
0.2
\end{array}
\quad \text{Total of three decimal places}
$$

Step 3: Mark off three decimal places in product.

New decimal $\longrightarrow$ .2 0 6

The answer is 0.206.

REMEMBER

When the number of places to be marked off goes beyond the numbers in the product, add a zero in each place.

RULE

To multiply a decimal fraction by 10,000, 1000, and so on, move the decimal to the *right* as many places as there are zeros in the multiplier.

EXAMPLE: Multiply 0.02 by 100. 100 has two zeros. Write 0.02, and move the decimal to the right two places.

0 0 2.

The answer is 2.0.

RULE

To multiply a decimal fraction by 0.1, 0.01, 0.001, and so on, move the decimal to the *left* as many places as there are decimal places in the multiplier.

EXAMPLE: Multiply 1.2 × 0.1; 0.1 has one decimal place. Write 1.2, and move the decimal to the left one place.

0. 1 2

The answer is 0.12.

REMEMBER

If the decimal must be moved farther than there are numbers, add a zero for each decimal place.

PRACTICE PROBLEMS—MULTIPLICATION OF DECIMAL FRACTIONS

Multiply the following decimal fractions:

1.	4.543	3.	1.793	5.	13.85
	× 0.17		× 1.2		× 1.08

2.	5.18	4.	0.7388	6.	49.034
	× 0.39		× 0.56		× 0.69

7.   0.326
   $\times$ 0.03

8.   0.4372
   $\times$ 0.61

9.   5.0499
   $\times$ 2.013

10.   24.678
   $\times$ 1.35

11.   1.9
   $\times$4.62

12.   7.253
   $\times$0.405

13.   11.02
   $\times$ 0.26

14.   5.79
   $\times$0.34

15.   0.467
   $\times$0.246

In the following problems, multiply by moving the decimal:

16. 14.5×10

17. 71.82×100

18. 14.26×10

19. 8.32×1000

20. 23.89×100

21. 12.26×10

22. 84.08×100

23. 18.53×1000

24. 26.7×100

25. 43.36×10

26. 32.216×1000

27. 4.27×100

28. 12.12×1000

29. 19.47×100

30. 6.10×10

31. 35.62×0.1

32. 16.43×0.01

33. 28.6×0.001

34. 18.47×0.001

35. 2.79×0.01

36. 0.45×0.1

37. 53.06×0.01

38. 8.27×0.001

39. 63.47×0.1

40. 47.7×0.001

41. 6.27×0.01

42. 0.98×0.1

43. 38.17×0.01

44. 26.94×0.1

45. 106.7×0.001

46. In a hospital gift shop, candy sells for $3.25 per lb. How much will 3.5 lb cost?

47. It takes 4.75 cups of water to dilute one container of nutritional supplement. How much water is needed to dilute three containers?

48. A patient pays $5.79 per day for medication. How much will he pay for 10 days?

49. What is 10 percent (0.10) of 85.930?

50. A package of transparent dressing costs $0.85. How much will 100 packages cost?

Division of Decimal Fractions

STEPS

To divide a *decimal* by a *whole number:*

1. Write the problem as usual.
2. Place a decimal on the quotient line directly above the decimal in the dividend.
3. Find the quotient.

Terms
2 ⟵ Quotient
Divisor ⟶ 5 $\overline{)10}$ ⟵ Dividend

EXAMPLE: Divide 0.1 by 25.

$$\begin{array}{r} 0.004 \\ 25\overline{)0.100} \\ \underline{100} \end{array}$$

The answer is 0.004.

STEPS

To divide a *whole number or a decimal fraction by a decimal fraction:*

1. Move the decimal in the divisor to the right until the divisor becomes a whole number.

2. Move the decimal in the dividend to the right as many places as you moved the decimal in the divisor.

3. Place the decimal on the quotient line directly above the new decimal in the dividend.

4. Divide as usual.

EXAMPLE: Divide 0.125 by 0.5.

↑   ↑

Dividend   Divisor

Decimal in quotient above decimal in dividend

↓

$$0\,5. \overline{)\,0\,1\,.2\,5}$$

Decimal moved one place   Decimal moved one
to make a whole number   place

Now the problem is:

$$
\begin{array}{r}
0.25 \\
5\,\overline{)\,1.25} \\
\underline{1\,0} \\
25 \\
\underline{25} \\
\end{array}
$$

The answer is 0.25.

RULE

To divide a decimal by 10, 100, 1000, and so on, move the decimal to the *left* as many places as there are zeros in the divisor.

EXAMPLE: Divide 0.05 by 1000.
Because 1000 has three zeros, move the decimal point three places to the *left.*

$$0.\,0\,0\,0\,0\,5$$

The answer is 0.00005.

RULE

> *To divide a decimal by 0.1, 0.01, 0.001, and so on,* move the decimal to the *right* as many places as there are decimal places in the divisor.

EXAMPLE: Divide 0.56 by 0.1.

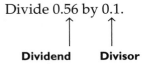

Dividend   Divisor

Because 0.1 has one decimal place, move the decimal one place to the *right.*

$$0\,5.6$$

The answer is 5.6.

PRACTICE PROBLEMS—DIVISION OF DECIMAL FRACTIONS

Carry out the following divisions to three places:

1. 0.6 ÷ 0.01	**6.** 64.926 ÷ 0.03	**11.** 170.01 ÷ 5.52
2. 55.120 ÷ 0.6	**7.** 39.364 ÷ 1.25	**12.** 250.61 ÷ 48.25
3. 76.02 ÷ 8.2	**8.** 51.267 ÷ 7.902	**13.** 74.025 ÷ 8.3
4. 135.500 ÷ 0.53	**9.** 2.81 ÷ 0.2	**14.** 54.728 ÷ 45.8
5. 67.05 ÷ 9.2	**10.** 32.224 ÷ 0.825	**15.** 26.749 ÷ 7.69

Divide the following problems by moving the decimal:

16. 0.93 ÷ 10	**19.** 6.07 ÷ 1000	**22.** 14.1 ÷ 10
17. 26.4 ÷ 100	**20.** 34 ÷ 100	**23.** 26.05 ÷ 100
18. 0.5 ÷ 1000	**21.** 8.7 ÷ 10	**24.** 14.9 ÷ 1000

25. $38.4 \div 100$

26. $26.35 \div 1000$

27. $138.5 \div 10$

28. $16.47 \div 1000$

29. $0.26 \div 100$

30. $7.19 \div 10$

31. $23.1 \div 0.1$

32. $85.6 \div 0.01$

33. $0.56 \div 0.001$

34. $64.2 \div 0.001$

35. $74.56 \div 0.01$

36. $85.1 \div 0.1$

37. $2.49 \div 0.01$

38. $13.54 \div 0.001$

39. $4.07 \div 0.1$

40. $0.64 \div 0.001$

41. $18.84 \div 0.01$

42. $9.17 \div 0.1$

43. $167.48 \div 0.01$

44. $35.9 \div 0.1$

45. $236.08 \div 0.001$

46. Mr. Brown bought 17.4 gal of gas and then drove 251.8 miles. How many miles to the gallon did he get?

47. Mrs. Stevens bought a ham for $6.59. The ham was sold at $1.19 per lb. How many lb of ham did Mrs. Stevens buy?

48. Tom wants a stereo set that costs $150.59. He earns $7.50 per week for doing household chores. How many weeks will he have to work to earn enough to buy the stereo?

49. Mr. Smith paints birdhouses. He uses 0.35 pt of paint on each house. How many birdhouses can he paint with 29.4 pt of paint?

50. Mr. Adams drove 1084.6 mi on his vacation. He averaged 271.1 mi per day. How many days was he gone?

Conversion of Fractions

STEPS

To change a numerical fraction to a decimal fraction, divide the denominator into the numerator.

EXAMPLE: Change $\frac{5}{10}$ to a decimal fraction.

$$\begin{array}{r} 0.5 \\ 10\overline{\smash{)}5.0} \\ \underline{5\ 0} \end{array} \qquad \frac{5}{10} = \mathbf{0.5}$$

PRACTICE PROBLEMS—CONVERSION OF FRACTIONS

Change the following numerical fractions to decimal fractions:

1. $\frac{3}{4}$ 4. $\frac{1}{150}$ 7. $\frac{1}{300}$ 10. $\frac{7}{8}$

2. $\frac{5}{7}$ 5. $\frac{11}{16}$ 8. $\frac{16}{20}$ 11. $\frac{1}{60}$

3. $\frac{12}{15}$ 6. $\frac{13}{20}$ 9. $\frac{5}{35}$ 12. $\frac{5}{9}$

STEPS

To change a decimal fraction to a numerical fraction, proceed as follows:

1. The number of decimal places determines the denominator —one place is 10, two places 100, and so on.

2. The number (drop the decimal) becomes the numerator.

3. Reduce to lowest terms.

EXAMPLE: Change 0.75 to a numerical fraction.
There are two decimal places, so the denominator is 100. Drop the decimal, and the numerator is 75.

$$0.75 = \frac{75}{100} \qquad (\tfrac{3}{4} \text{ in lowest terms})$$

PRACTICE PROBLEMS—CONVERSION OF DECIMAL FRACTIONS TO NUMERICAL FRACTIONS

Change the following decimal fractions to numerical fractions:

1. 0.2	**4.** 0.039	**7.** 0.50	**10.** 0.125
2. 0.11	**5.** 0.650	**8.** 0.25	**11.** 0.66
3. 0.36	**6.** 0.75	**9.** 0.938	**12.** 0.7

Percents

RULE

> The word *percent* literally means "part of 100." The term 15% means 15 parts of 100, or $\frac{15}{100}$. When you see a percent symbol, think of a fraction in which the denominator is 100.

EXAMPLE: Express 25% as a numerical fraction.

Step 1: Write 25 as the numerator.
Step 2: Write 100 as the denominator.
Step 3: Drop the % symbol.

25% is the same as $\frac{25}{100}$.

CHANGE PERCENT TO DECIMAL FRACTION

STEPS

To change a number expressed as a percent to a decimal fraction, divide the number by 100. This will move the decimal two places to the *left*. Drop the percent symbol.

EXAMPLE: Change 35% to a decimal fraction.

Step 1: Divide 35 by 100.

$$
\begin{array}{r}
.35 \\
100\overline{\smash{)}35.00} \\
\underline{30\ 0} \\
5\ 00 \\
\underline{5\ 00}
\end{array}
$$

Step 2: Drop the percent symbol.
35% is 0.35.

CHANGE DECIMAL FRACTION TO PERCENT

STEPS

To change a decimal fraction to a percent, remove the decimal by multiplying the number by 100 and adding a percent symbol.

EXAMPLE: Change 0.12 to a percent.

Step 1: Drop the decimal by multiplying .12 by 100.

$$0.12 \times 100 = 12$$

Step 2: Add the percent symbol.
0.12 is 12%.

CHANGE NUMERICAL FRACTION TO PERCENT

STEPS

To change a numerical fraction to a percent, divide the denominator into the numerator, multiply by 100, and add the percent symbol.

EXAMPLE: Change $\frac{3}{4}$ to a percent.

Step 1. Divide 3 by 4.

$$
\begin{array}{r}
0.75 \\
4\overline{)\ 3.00} \\
\underline{2\,8} \\
20 \\
\underline{20}
\end{array}
$$

Step 2. Multiply 0.75 by 100 = 75.
Step 3. Add the percent symbol.

$\frac{3}{4}$ is 75%.

PRACTICE PROBLEMS—PERCENT

Change to a numerical fraction:

1. 3%   **2.** 17%   **3.** 38%   **4.** 52%

Change to a decimal fraction:

5. 15%	**6.** 27%	**7.** 49%	**8.** 78%

Change to a percent:

9. 0.08	**11.** 0.32	**13.** $\frac{1}{4}$	**15.** $\frac{2}{3}$
10. 0.19	**12.** 0.64	**14.** $\frac{1}{2}$	**16.** $\frac{5}{8}$

ANSWERS
Addition of Decimal Fractions (pp. 20–21)

1. 32.56	**10.** 9.2015	**19.** 77.38
2. 207.58	**11.** 28.21	**20.** 210.783
3. 70.30	**12.** 16.17	**21.** $6.81
4. 839.23	**13.** 49.513	**22.** 67.6
5. 203.36	**14.** 148.72	**23.** $62,879.59
6. 974.9	**15.** 29.537	**24.** 671.58
7. 1.902	**16.** 56.13	**25.** 3745.912
8. 56.0092	**17.** 151.397	
9. 29.62	**18.** 62.676	

Subtraction of Decimal Fractions (pp. 22–23)

1. 2.1	**8.** 32.731	**15.** 5.1259	**22.** $1701.78
2. 2.21	**9.** 1.982	**16.** 0.5373	**23.** 494.22
3. 25.5	**10.** 7.09981	**17.** 0.00047	**24.** $47.34
4. 8.055	**11.** 11.0761	**18.** 10.204	**25.** 48
5. 16.96	**12.** 1.0904	**19.** 2.2188	
6. 19.85	**13.** 62.74	**20.** 2.102	
7. 3.952	**14.** 104.099	**21.** 4.66	

Multiplication of Decimal Fractions (p. 24–26)

These answers are rounded off to three places.

1. 0.772	**14.** 1.969	**27.** 427	**40.** 0.048
2. 2.020	**15.** 0.115	**28.** 12,120	**41.** 0.063
3. 2.152	**16.** 145	**29.** 1947	**42.** 0.098
4. 0.414	**17.** 7182	**30.** 61	**43.** 0.382
5. 14.958	**18.** 142.6	**31.** 3.562	**44.** 2.694
6. 33.833	**19.** 8320	**32.** 0.164	**45.** 0.107
7. 0.010	**20.** 2389	**33.** 0.029	**46.** $11.38
8. 0.267	**21.** 122.6	**34.** 0.018	**47.** 14.25
9. 10.165	**22.** 8408	**35.** 0.028	**48.** $57.90
10. 33.315	**23.** 18,530	**36.** 0.045	**49.** 8.593
11. 8.778	**24.** 2670	**37.** 0.531	**50.** $85.00
12. 2.937	**25.** 433.6	**38.** 0.008	
13. 2.865	**26.** 32,216	**39.** 6.347	

Division of Decimal Fractions (p. 28–29)

1. 60	**14.** 1.195	**27.** 13.85	**40.** 640
2. 91.867	**15.** 3.478	**28.** 0.01647	**41.** 1884
3. 9.271	**16.** 0.093	**29.** 0.0026	**42.** 91.7
4. 255.660	**17.** 0.264	**30.** 0.719	**43.** 16,748
5. 7.288	**18.** 0.0005	**31.** 231	**44.** 359
6. 2164.2	**19.** 0.00607	**32.** 8560	**45.** 236,080
7. 31.491	**20.** 0.34	**33.** 560	**46.** 14.471
8. 6.488	**21.** 0.87	**34.** 64,200	**47.** 5.538
9. 14.050	**22.** 1.41	**35.** 7456	**48.** 20.08
10. 39.059	**23.** 0.2605	**36.** 851	**49.** 84
11. 30.799	**24.** 0.0149	**37.** 249	**50.** 4
12. 5.194	**25.** 0.384	**38.** 13,540	
13. 8.919	**26.** 0.02635	**39.** 40.7	

Conversion of Fractions (p. 30)

1. 0.75	**4.** 0.007	**7.** 0.003	**10.** 0.88
2. 0.71	**5.** 0.69	**8.** 0.8	**11.** 0.02
3. 0.8	**6.** 0.65	**9.** 0.14	**12.** 0.56

Conversion of Decimal Fractions to Numerical Fractions (p. 31)

1. $\frac{2}{10}$ or $\frac{1}{5}$

2. $\frac{11}{100}$

3. $\frac{36}{100}$ or $\frac{9}{25}$

4. $\frac{39}{1000}$

5. $\frac{65}{100}$ or $\frac{13}{20}$

6. $\frac{75}{100}$ or $\frac{3}{4}$

7. $\frac{50}{100}$ or $\frac{1}{2}$

8. $\frac{25}{100}$ or $\frac{1}{4}$

9. $\frac{938}{1000}$ or $\frac{469}{500}$

10. $\frac{125}{1000}$ or $\frac{1}{8}$

11. $\frac{66}{100}$ or $\frac{33}{50}$

12. $\frac{7}{10}$

Percent (p. 32–33)

1. $\frac{3}{100}$

2. $\frac{17}{100}$

3. $\frac{38}{100}$

4. $\frac{52}{100}$

5. 0.15

6. 0.27

7. 0.49

8. 0.78

9. 8%

10. 19%

11. 32%

12. 64%

13. 25%

14. 50%

15. 67%

16. 6%

CHAPTER 3

Ratio and Proportion

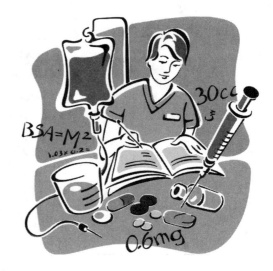

A *ratio* is a mathematical expression that compares two numbers by division. The division symbol can be written as −, /, or :. The ratio 2/3 is read "2 is to 3."

EXAMPLE: Write *7 is to 15* as a ratio.

$$\frac{7}{15}, 7/15, \text{ or } 7{:}15$$

REMEMBER

> A ratio can be reduced to lowest terms and still have the same value.

A *proportion* is a statement that says two ratios are equal. $1/2 = 5/10$ is a proportion. It can also be written using colons—$1:2::5:10$. When expressed this way, the double colon :: stands for the symbol =, and is read, "as." The proportion $1:2::5:10$ is read, "One is to two as five is to ten."

In a proportion, the terms have names. The *extremes* are the two outside terms, and the *means* are the two inside terms.

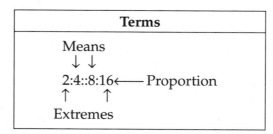

RULE

> In a proportion, the product of the means is equal to the product of the extremes.

Many times we know only three terms of a proportion. The term we do not know is the "unknown," and in this book is labeled X.

Solving for the "Unknown"

> **STEPS**
>
> **1.** Multiply the extremes and multiply the means.
>
> **2.** Set their products equal.
>
> **3.** Divide both sides of the equation by the number to the left of X.

EXAMPLE: Solve $2 : 3 : : X : 6$

Step 1: Multiply the extremes: $2 \times 6 = 12$. Multiply the means: $3 \times X = 3X$.

Step 2: Set their products equal: $3X = 12$.

Step 3: Divide both sides of the equation by the number to the left of X. In this case, 3 is the number.

$$\frac{3X}{3} = \frac{12}{3}$$

$$\frac{\overset{1}{\cancel{3X}}}{\underset{1}{\cancel{3}}} = \frac{\overset{4}{\cancel{12}}}{\underset{1}{\cancel{3}}}$$

$$X = \mathbf{4}$$

To see if 4 is the correct answer, use 4 in the problem in place of X. The products of the means and extremes should be equal.

$$2 : 3 : : 4 : 6 \qquad 2 \times 6 = 12$$
$$3 \times 4 = 12$$

$12 = 12$, so 4 is the correct answer.

EXAMPLE: Solve $6 : 10X : : 3 : 15$.

Multiply means.

6:10X::3:15

Multiply extremes.

$30X = 90$ **Set their products equal**

$\dfrac{30X}{30} = \dfrac{90}{30}$ **Divide both sides by the number to the left of X**

$X = \mathbf{3}$

EXAMPLE: Consider this problem. Six thermometers cost $2. How many thermometers can be purchased for $4?

REMEMBER

> When setting up a proportion, the terms of the second ratio must be written in the same order as the terms of the first ratio.

Write the first ratio as stated in the problem. This is what is given, or what is known, and is termed the *known equivalent*.

In this example, the first ratio is 6 thermometers: $2. The second ratio must be in the same order, that is, thermometers: $.

The second ratio is X thermometers : $4. Now we can write the entire proportion:

$$6 \text{ thermometers} : \$2 :: X \text{ thermometers} : \$4$$

Now the proportion can be solved. (At this point we may drop all labels except for X. *Always keep X labeled.*)

$$6 : 2 :: X \text{ thermometers} : 4$$

(extremes) $6 \times 4 = 24$

(means) $2 \times X \text{ thermometers} = 2X \text{ thermometers}$
$2X \text{ thermometers} = 24$

$$\frac{^1\cancel{2}X \text{ thermometers}}{\cancel{2}_{\,1}} = \frac{\cancel{24}^{\,12}}{\cancel{2}_{\,1}}$$

$$X = \textbf{12 thermometers}$$

Remember that a proportion can also be written in this format:

$$\frac{2}{10} = \frac{X}{20}$$

It is read as 2 is to 10 as X is to 20.

RULE

> To solve this type of proportion, use *cross-multiplication*; that is, multiply across the equal sign.

EXAMPLE: To solve

$$\frac{2}{10} = \frac{X}{20}$$

use these steps:
1. Multiply X and the number diagonally opposite to X.

$$\frac{2}{10} \nearrow \frac{X}{20} \rightarrow \textbf{10 X}$$

2. Multiply the other two numbers.

$$\frac{2}{10} \searrow \frac{X}{20} \rightarrow \textbf{40}$$

3. Set the products equal, and solve for X.

$$10X = 40$$

$$\frac{^{1}\cancel{10}X}{\cancel{10}_{1}} = \frac{\cancel{40}^{4}}{\cancel{10}_{1}}$$

$$X = 4$$

Is X really 4? Prove it by substituting 4 for X in the original problem.

$$\frac{2}{10} = \frac{4}{20}$$

Then cross-multiply.

$$\frac{2}{10} \diagup\!\!\!\!\diagdown \frac{4}{20}$$

$$40 = \mathbf{40}$$

X is indeed 4.

EXAMPLE: Consider this problem: Ten children can ride in one van. How many children can ride in three vans? The problem tells you how many children can ride in one van. This information is the *known equivalent* and is used for the first ratio. Set up the second ratio in the same order as the first.

$$\frac{10 \text{ children}}{1 \text{ van}} = \frac{X \text{ children}}{3 \text{ vans}}$$

(Drop all labels except for X.) Cross-multiply and solve for X.

$$\frac{10}{1} \diagup\!\!\!\!\diagdown \frac{X \text{ children}}{3}$$

$$X = \mathbf{30 \text{ children}}$$

REMEMBER

When you solve problems using ratio and proportion, you may set up the problem as:

$$2:10::4:X \text{ or } \frac{2}{10} = \frac{4}{X}$$

Either format is acceptable.

PRACTICE PROBLEMS—RATIO AND PROPORTION

1. $1 : 2 :: X : 6$

2. $3 : 5 :: X : 4$

3. $7 : 10 :: X : 3$

4. $X : 15 :: 1 : 3$

5. $7 : 20 :: X : 10$

6. $25 : 100 :: 100 : X$

7. $4 : 25 :: 15 : X$

8. $11 : 16 :: X : 8$

9. $2 : 9 :: X : 3$

10. $3 : X :: 14 : 20$

11. $3 : 2 :: X : 4$

12. $5 : 6 :: 7 : X$

13. $7 : 10 :: X : 25$

14. $2 : 3 :: X : 18$

15. $5 : 12 :: X : 8$

16. $9 : 10 :: X : 30$

17. $7 : 8 :: X : 24$

18. $4 : 5 :: X : 35$

19. $\frac{2}{5} : 1 :: \frac{3}{10} : X$

20. $\frac{5}{8} : 2 :: \frac{1}{2} : X$

21. $X : \frac{4}{6} :: 5 : \frac{1}{2}$

22. $\frac{7}{20} : 10 :: \frac{5}{10} : X$

23. $\frac{4}{25} : 5 :: \frac{7}{15} : X$

24. $\frac{11}{16} : X :: \frac{5}{8} : 4$

25. $\frac{9}{16} : X :: \frac{1}{2} : 8$

26. $\frac{3}{14} : X :: \frac{5}{9} : 11$

27. $\frac{2}{5} : 12 :: 2\frac{2}{5} : X$

28. $\frac{12}{15} : X :: \frac{2}{25} : 15$

29. $X : \frac{5}{8} :: 4\frac{1}{2} : 9$

30. $\frac{11}{14} : X :: 3\frac{4}{6} : 5$

31. $4\frac{5}{6} : X :: \frac{15}{16} : 21$

32. $X : \frac{3}{4} :: 2\frac{2}{3} : 15$

33. $3\frac{1}{2} : X :: 12 : \frac{3}{4}$

34. $X : 2\frac{3}{4} :: 24 : \frac{5}{6}$

35. $\frac{7}{10} : 11 :: \frac{2}{3} : X$

36. $2\frac{7}{8} : X :: \frac{5}{12} : 14$

37. $3.7 : X :: 5.8 : 10$

38. $10.9 : 15 :: 24.6 : X$

39. $50.4 : 100 :: X : 12.2$

40. $5.34 : X :: 3.5 : 9$

41. $3.7 : X :: 5.8 : 7$

42. $X : 12.3 :: 10.9 : 30$

43. $4.6 : 7.9 :: X : 18$

44. $1.5 : 15 :: X : 2.5$

45. $1.25 : X :: 3.5 : 10$

46. $7.3 : 40 :: 8.5 : X$

47. $0.1 : X :: 100 : 10$

48. $0.5X : 3 :: 0.7 : 0.28$

49. $3.4 : X :: 6.7 : 9$

50. $X : 5.8 :: 3.4 : 7$

51. $7.7 : 1.4 :: X : 63$

52. $0.61 : X :: 0.2 : 0.4$

53. $0.1 : 0.3 :: 8 : X$

54. $2.6X : 15 :: 4.1 : 10$

55. $\frac{1}{2} = \frac{X}{10}$

56. $\frac{3}{5} = \frac{4}{X}$

57. $\frac{2}{3} = \frac{X}{15}$

58. $\frac{X}{11} = \frac{4}{13}$

59. $\frac{5}{X} = \frac{25}{100}$

60. $\frac{15}{20} = \frac{X}{15}$

61. $\frac{32}{64} = \frac{100}{X}$

62. $\frac{17}{68} = \frac{20}{X}$

63. $\frac{X}{10} = \frac{16}{72}$

64. $\frac{9}{X} = \frac{36}{3}$

65. $\frac{X}{100} = \frac{25}{1000}$

66. $\frac{2}{4} = \frac{X}{30}$

67. $\frac{1}{5} = \frac{X}{35}$

68. $\frac{14}{9} = \frac{35}{X}$

69. $\frac{X}{17} = \frac{35}{10}$

70. $\frac{11}{18} = \frac{X}{36}$

71. $\frac{8}{64} = \frac{15}{X}$

72. $\frac{X}{12} = \frac{6}{18}$

73. $\frac{\frac{1}{2}}{X} = \frac{8}{\frac{2}{3}}$

74. $\frac{X}{\frac{1}{3}} = \frac{\frac{1}{7}}{7}$

75. $\frac{\frac{14}{5}}{X} = \frac{2}{\frac{1}{7}}$

76. $\frac{\frac{3}{2}}{X} = \frac{\frac{2}{5}}{10}$

77. $\frac{X}{\frac{1}{5}} = \frac{16}{13}$

78. $\frac{\frac{18}{9}}{2} = \frac{\frac{1}{9}}{X}$

79. $\frac{4}{\frac{1}{2}} = \frac{X}{\frac{14}{28}}$

80. $\frac{\frac{3}{5}X}{10} = \frac{15}{16}$

81. $\frac{4\frac{2}{3}}{X} = \frac{3\frac{1}{5}}{9}$

82. $\frac{X}{6\frac{1}{2}} = \frac{2}{13}$

83. $\frac{\frac{1}{16}}{\frac{1}{10}} = \frac{X}{\frac{1}{2}}$

84. $\frac{\frac{3}{3}}{\frac{3}{8}} = \frac{X}{4\frac{1}{4}}$

85. $\dfrac{\frac{1}{2}}{2} = \dfrac{5\frac{2}{3}}{X}$

86. $\dfrac{6X}{\frac{2}{7}} = \dfrac{42}{\frac{1}{14}}$

87. $\dfrac{\frac{6}{49}}{1} = \dfrac{\frac{8}{15}}{X}$

88. $\dfrac{46}{X} = \dfrac{\frac{1}{2}}{\frac{1}{10}}$

89. $\dfrac{2\frac{1}{3}}{3} = \dfrac{X}{15}$

90. $\dfrac{X}{3\frac{1}{2}} = \dfrac{\frac{2}{7}}{20}$

91. $\dfrac{0.3}{0.6} = \dfrac{0.4}{X}$

92. $\dfrac{1.7}{X} = \dfrac{8.2}{0.8}$

93. $\dfrac{1.1}{X} = \dfrac{0.6}{0.5}$

94. $\dfrac{X}{0.35} = \dfrac{0.5}{10}$

95. $\dfrac{0.41}{0.26} = \dfrac{X}{0.67}$

96. $\dfrac{0.34}{0.7} = \dfrac{19}{X}$

97. $\dfrac{1.8}{0.47} = \dfrac{X}{1.3}$

98. $\dfrac{X}{0.54} = \dfrac{3.6}{15}$

99. $\dfrac{0.28}{0.11} = \dfrac{5}{16X}$

100. $\dfrac{X}{0.29} = \dfrac{64}{73}$

101. $\dfrac{0.8}{0.9} = \dfrac{0.7}{X}$

102. $\dfrac{12.6}{X} = \dfrac{15}{18}$

103. $\dfrac{0.11}{0.28} = \dfrac{X}{0.43}$

104. $\dfrac{4.7}{X} = \dfrac{6.4}{19}$

105. $\dfrac{35.9}{10} = \dfrac{X}{100}$

106. $\dfrac{0.1}{0.001} = \dfrac{X}{0.001}$

107. $\dfrac{9.17}{18} = \dfrac{X}{4.2}$

108. $\dfrac{1000\,X}{100} = \dfrac{0.01}{0.001}$

Use ratio and proportion to solve these word problems. Be sure to identify the known equivalent and write it as the first ratio.

109. To make one cake, use $2\frac{3}{4}$ cups flour. How much flour is needed to make three cakes?

110. Five yd of paper tape costs $15.35. How much does 1 yd cost?

111. Bob traveled 369 mi in one day on a bus trip. How many mi could he travel in $9\frac{1}{2}$ days?

112. Three peaches sell for $1. How many can you buy for $10?

113. An antiseptic is sold for $3.59 per 50 oz. How much is paid per oz?

114. One assembly line worker can assemble $7\frac{1}{2}$ model cars per hour. How many cars could nine workers produce per hour?

115. Mrs. Smith bought a 20 lb turkey for $17.96. How much did she pay per lb?

116. Brand *A* peaches sell for $0.79 per 20 oz. Brand *B* peaches are $1.85 for 64 oz. Which is the better buy?

117. If Ed must work 5 days to earn $259.53, how many days would he have to work to earn $4412.01?

118. Patricia can work an average of 50 math problems in one hour. How many problems can she work in 12 minutes?

ANSWERS

Ratio and Proportion (pp. 40–43)

1. 3	**10.** 4.286	**19.** $\frac{3}{4}$	**28.** 150
2. 2.4	**11.** 6	**20.** $1\frac{3}{5}$	**29.** $\frac{5}{16}$
3. 2.1	**12.** 8.4	**21.** $6\frac{2}{3}$	**30.** $1\frac{1}{14}$
4. 5	**13.** 17.5	**22.** $14\frac{2}{7}$	**31.** 108.27
5. 3.5	**14.** 12	**23.** $14\frac{7}{12}$	**32.** $\frac{2}{15}$
6. 400	**15.** 3.333	**24.** $4\frac{2}{5}$	**33.** $\frac{7}{32}$
7. 93.75	**16.** 27	**25.** 9	**34.** $79\frac{1}{5}$
8. 5.5	**17.** 21	**26.** $4\frac{17}{70}$	**35.** 10.476
9. 0.667	**18.** 28	**27.** 72	**36.** $96\frac{3}{5}$

37. 6.379

38. 33.853

39. 6.1488

40. 13.731

41. 4.466

42. 4.469

43. 10.481

44. 0.25

45. 3.571

46. 46.575

47. 0.01

48. 15

49. 4.567

50. 2.817

51. 346.5

52. 1.22

53. 24

54. 2.365

55. 5

56. $6\frac{2}{3}$

57. 10

58. $3\frac{5}{13}$

59. 20

60. $11\frac{1}{4}$

61. 200

62. 80

63. $2\frac{2}{10}$

64. $\frac{3}{4}$

65. $2\frac{1}{2}$

66. 15

67. 7

68. $22\frac{1}{2}$

69. $59\frac{1}{2}$

70. 22

71. 120

72. 4

73. $\frac{1}{24}$

74. $\frac{1}{147}$

75. $\frac{1}{5}$

76. $37\frac{1}{2}$

77. $\frac{16}{65}$

78. $\frac{1}{9}$

79. 4

80. $15\frac{5}{8}$

81. $13\frac{1}{8}$

82. 1

83. $\frac{5}{16}$

84. 34

85. $22\frac{2}{3}$

86. 28

87. $4\frac{16}{45}$

88. $9\frac{1}{5}$

89. $11\frac{2}{3}$

90. $\frac{1}{20}$

91. 0.8

92. 0.166

93. 0.917

94. 0.0175

95. 1.057

96. 39.118

97. 4.979

98. 0.13

99. 0.123

100. 0.254

101. 0.788

102. 15.12

103. 0.168

104. 13.953

105. 359

106. 0.1

107. 2.14

108. 1

109. $8\frac{1}{4}$

110. $3.07

111. 3505.5

112. 30

113. $0.07

114. 67.5

115. $0.90

116. Brand B

117. 85

118. 10

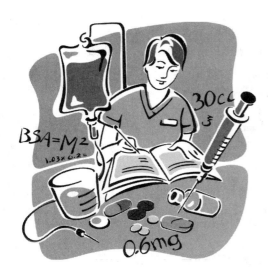

CHAPTER 4

Roman Numerals

Roman numerals are used to express numerical value in the apothecary system of measurement (Chapter 6). Several letters—$\overline{ss}$, i, v, x, l, c, d, m—are used separately or in combination to express all numbers in the Roman system. The smaller Roman numerals ($\overline{ss}$, i, v, x) are more commonly used. The larger numerals are included as additional information.

$$\overline{ss} = \tfrac{1}{2}$$
$$i = 1$$
$$v = 5$$
$$x = 10$$
$$l = 50$$
$$c = 100$$
$$d = 500$$
$$m = 1000$$

REMEMBER	
	It is rare to use numbers larger than 45 in the apothecary system.

RULE	
	All numbers are written in terms of addition, subtraction, or both. If a letter of lesser value precedes a larger letter (such as iv—i = one, v = five), then you subtract. The Roman numeral iv means subtract one from five, which is four. If a letter of lesser or equal value follows another letter, then you add. In Roman numerals, xx means 10 + 10 and is read as 20.

EXAMPLE: Let's look at a more difficult number: xlviii$\overline{ss}$.

xl means $50 - 10 = $ **40**
viii means $5 + 3 = $ **8**
$\overline{ss}$ means $\frac{1}{2}$
xlviii$\overline{ss}$ $= $ **$48\frac{1}{2}$**

EXAMPLE: Write 33 in Roman numerals.

30 is **10 + 10 + 10 or xxx**
3 is **1 + 1 + 1 or iii**
33 is **xxxiii**

PRACTICE PROBLEMS—EXPRESSING ARABIC NUMERALS IN ROMAN NUMERALS

Express the following Arabic numerals in Roman numerals:

1. $1\frac{1}{2}$ 6. 21   11. 3   16. $23\frac{1}{2}$

2. 5   7. 25   12. $7\frac{1}{2}$ 17. 27

3. 9   8. 29   13. 11   18. 31

4. $13\frac{1}{2}$ 9. $33\frac{1}{2}$ 14. 15   19. $35\frac{1}{2}$

5. 17   10. 39   15. 19   20. 41

PRACTICE PROBLEMS—CHANGING ROMAN NUMERALS TO ARABIC NUMERALS

Change these Roman numerals to Arabic numerals:

1. ii   3. x   5. xviii   7. xxviii

2. vi   4. xiv$\overline{ss}$ 6. xxii   8. xxxiv

9. xl   **12.** viii$\overline{ss}$ **15.** xx$\overline{ss}$ **18.** xxxvi$\overline{ss}$

10. xliv   **13.** xii   **16.** xxvi$\overline{ss}$ **19.** xlii

11. iv$\overline{ss}$ **14.** xvi   **17.** xxxii   **20.** xlv

---

ANSWERS

Expressing Arabic Numerals in Roman Numerals (pp. 46)

1. iss	**6.** xxi	**11.** iii	**16.** xxiii$\overline{ss}$
2. v	**7.** xxv	**12.** vii$\overline{ss}$	**17.** xxvii
3. ix	**8.** xxix	**13.** xi	**18.** xxxi
4. xiii$\overline{ss}$	**9.** xxxiii$\overline{ss}$	**14.** xv	**19.** xxxv$\overline{ss}$
5. xvii	**10.** xxxix	**15.** xix	**20.** xli

Changing Roman Numerals to Arabic Numerals (pp. 46–47)

1. 2	**6.** 22	**11.** $4\frac{1}{2}$	**16.** $26\frac{1}{2}$
2. 6	**7.** 28	**12.** $8\frac{1}{2}$	**17.** 32
3. 10	**8.** 34	**13.** 12	**18.** $36\frac{1}{2}$
4. $14\frac{1}{2}$	**9.** 40	**14.** 16	**19.** 42
5. 18	**10.** 44	**15.** $20\frac{1}{2}$	**20.** 45

UNIT 1

Comprehensive Test

Add:

1. $\frac{2}{7} + \frac{3}{8} + \frac{1}{4}$

5. $5\frac{2}{3} + 7\frac{3}{12} + 10\frac{1}{4}$

2. $\frac{1}{16} + \frac{2}{4} + \frac{7}{8}$

6. $3\frac{12}{16} + 4\frac{5}{64} + 11\frac{3}{8}$

3. $\frac{1}{2} + \frac{5}{6} + \frac{2}{7}$

7. $8\frac{3}{7} + 14\frac{7}{21} + 103$

4. $3\frac{1}{8} + 9\frac{4}{5} + 11\frac{3}{4}$

Subtract:

8. $\begin{array}{r} \frac{3}{4} \\ -\frac{3}{8} \\ \hline \end{array}$

10. $\begin{array}{r} \frac{2}{3} \\ -\frac{1}{4} \\ \hline \end{array}$

12. $\begin{array}{r} 11\frac{1}{2} \\ -9\frac{3}{8} \\ \hline \end{array}$

14. $\begin{array}{r} 18\frac{11}{16} \\ -6\frac{25}{64} \\ \hline \end{array}$

9. $\begin{array}{r} \frac{4}{5} \\ -\frac{1}{2} \\ \hline \end{array}$

11. $\begin{array}{r} \frac{5}{8} \\ -\frac{9}{16} \\ \hline \end{array}$

13. $\begin{array}{r} 15\frac{4}{5} \\ -7\frac{1}{3} \\ \hline \end{array}$

Multiply:

15. $\frac{3}{16} \times \frac{5}{8}$ **19.** $17\frac{1}{3} \times 14\frac{11}{16}$

16. $\frac{1}{2} \times \frac{2}{3} \times \frac{1}{4}$ **20.** $10\frac{15}{20} \times 7\frac{3}{4}$

17. $\frac{5}{6} \times \frac{5}{9}$ **21.** $5\frac{15}{18} \times 3\frac{3}{9} \times 7\frac{2}{3}$

18. $12\frac{4}{5} \times 11\frac{5}{6}$ **22.** $105 \times \frac{1}{150} \times 10\frac{1}{2}$

Divide:

23. $\frac{10}{14} \div \frac{19}{28}$ **26.** $9\frac{3}{4} \div \frac{1}{3}$ **29.** $12\frac{1}{4} \div 9\frac{1}{2}$

24. $\frac{5}{8} \div \frac{5}{6}$ **27.** $11 \div \frac{3}{16}$ **30.** $7\frac{4}{5} \div 11\frac{3}{8}$

25. $\frac{4}{5} \div \frac{2}{3}$ **28.** $24\frac{5}{7} \div 1\frac{3}{4}$

Add:

31. $23.28 + 3.5$ **35.** $23.47 + 0.236 + 15$

32. $0.25 + 46.05 + 10$ **36.** $4.6 + 0.14 + 63.46$

33. $0.07 + 3.6 + 2.15$ **37.** $3.47 + 53.52 + 243.6$

34. $634.24 + 0.19 + 0.34$

Subtract:

38. 4368
    − 3.06

40. 46.3
    − 0.025

42.   0.456
    −0.34

44. 42.38
    − 1.46

39. 43.26
    − 5.4

41. 3.27
    −0.35

43. 37.64
    − 0.037

Multiply:

45.   32.5
    ×47.8

47.   3.2
    ×0.478

49.   67.39
    ×240.19

51.   63.87
    × 0.768

46.   4.63
    ×23.37

48.   4.53
    ×0.001

50. 548.7
    × 65.93

52. 56.7
    ×80.02

Divide:

53. 34.42 ÷ 0.25

56. 53.65 ÷ 0.34

59. 256.43 ÷ 0.01

54. 46.37 ÷ 0.045

57. 100.2 ÷ 0.001

60. 347.67 ÷ 0.036

55. 27.43 ÷ 0.07

58. 242.65 ÷ 10

Solve:

61. $2 : 3 : : 10 : X$

62. $15 : 19 : : 27 : X$

63. $X : 27 : : 3 : 9$

64. $10 : X : : 25 : 50$

65. $100 : 1000 : : X : 100$

66. $\frac{4}{8} : \frac{3}{4} : : \frac{1}{16} : X$

67. $\frac{2}{3} : X : : \frac{5}{12} : \frac{3}{9}$

68. $X : \frac{1}{4} : : \frac{1}{2} : 2$

69. $\frac{2}{5} : 5 : : \frac{3}{10} : X$

70. $\frac{5}{24} : 10 : : X : 15$

71. $3.5 : X : : 5 : 20$

72. $10 : 2.5 : : X : 16$

73. $8.2 : 4.3 : : 2.5 : X$

74. $0.4 : 0.6 : : X : 100$

75. $1.5X : 5 : : 3.5 : 45$

76. $\frac{2}{6} = \frac{5}{X}$

77. $\frac{3}{X} = \frac{4}{9}$

78. $\frac{4}{12} = \frac{X}{18}$

79. $\frac{5}{40} = \frac{10}{X}$

80. $\frac{X}{7} = \frac{24}{35}$

81. $\dfrac{\frac{2}{3}}{X} = \dfrac{\frac{3}{4}}{\frac{5}{6}}$

82. $\dfrac{X}{\frac{4}{15}} = \dfrac{11}{\frac{3}{9}}$

83. $\dfrac{\frac{2}{5}}{X} = \dfrac{\frac{3}{10}}{15}$

84. $\dfrac{\frac{5}{24}}{48} = \dfrac{\frac{7}{16}}{X}$

85. $\dfrac{\frac{1}{3}}{9} = \dfrac{X}{18}$

86. $\dfrac{0.3}{0.9} = \dfrac{1.5}{X}$

87. $\dfrac{0.18}{0.36} = \dfrac{X}{100}$

88. $\dfrac{X}{0.27} = \dfrac{0.08}{0.32}$

89. $\dfrac{32.6}{X} = \dfrac{14}{3.7}$

90. $\dfrac{4.1}{5.6} = \dfrac{X}{33.7}$

Change to Roman Numerals:

91. $1\frac{1}{2}$

93. $32\frac{1}{2}$

95. 19

92. 16

94. 27

Change to Arabic Numerals:

96. iv$\overline{ss}$

98. xxxix

100. ix$\overline{ss}$

97. xi

99. xxii$\overline{ss}$

Change to Numerical Fractions:

101. 7%

102. 47%

103. 81%

Change to Decimal Fractions:

104. 6%

105. 32%

106. 95%

Change to Percentages:

107. 0.15

109. $\frac{1}{5}$

110. $\frac{1}{10}$

108. 0.73

ANSWERS

Unit 1: Comprehensive Test (pp. 48–52)

1. $\frac{51}{56}$

2. $1\frac{7}{16}$

3. $1\frac{13}{21}$

4. $24\frac{27}{40}$

5. $23\frac{1}{6}$

6. $19\frac{13}{64}$

7. $125\frac{16}{21}$

8. $\frac{3}{8}$

9. $\frac{3}{10}$

10. $\frac{5}{12}$

11. $\frac{1}{16}$

12. $2\frac{1}{8}$

13. $8\frac{7}{15}$

14. $12\frac{19}{64}$

15. $\frac{15}{128}$

16. $\frac{1}{12}$

17. $\frac{25}{54}$

18. $151\frac{7}{15}$

19. $254\frac{14}{24}$

20. $83\frac{5}{16}$

21. $149\frac{6}{81}$

22. $7\frac{21}{60}$

23. $1\frac{1}{19}$

24. $\frac{3}{4}$

25. $1\frac{1}{5}$

26. $29\frac{1}{4}$

27. $58\frac{2}{3}$

28. $14\frac{6}{49}$

29. $1\frac{11}{38}$

30. $\frac{312}{455}$

31. 26.78

32. 56.3

33. 5.82

34. 634.77

35. 38.706

36. 68.2

37. 300.59

38. 4364.94

39. 37.86

40. 46.275

41. 2.92

42. 0.116

43. 37.603

44. 40.92

45. 1553.5

46. 108.203

47. 1.5296

48. 0.00453

49. 16,186.404

50. 36,175.791

51. 49.052

52. 4537.134

53. 137.68

54. 1030.444

55. 391.857

56. 157.794

57. 100,200

58. 24.265

59. 25,643

60. 9657.5

61. 15

62. 34.2

63. 9

64. 20

65. 10

66. $\frac{3}{32}$

67. $\frac{8}{15}$

68. $\frac{1}{16}$

69. $3\frac{3}{4}$

70. $\frac{5}{16}$

71. 14

72. 64

73. 1.311

74. 66.666

75. 0.259

76. 15

77. 6.75 or $6\frac{3}{4}$

78. 6

79. 80

80. 4.8 or $4\frac{4}{5}$

81. $\frac{20}{27}$

82. 8.8

83. 20

84. 100.8

85. $\frac{2}{3}$

86. 4.5

87. 50

88. 0.0675

89. 8.616

90. 24.673

91. $\overline{\text{iss}}$

92. xvi

93. xxxii$\overline{\text{ss}}$

94. xxvii

95. xix

96. $4\frac{1}{2}$

97. 11

98. 39

99. $22\frac{1}{2}$

100. $9\frac{1}{2}$

101. $\frac{7}{100}$

102. $\frac{47}{100}$

103. $\frac{81}{100}$

104. 0.06

105. 0.32

106. 0.95

107. 15%

108. 73%

109. 20%

110. 10%

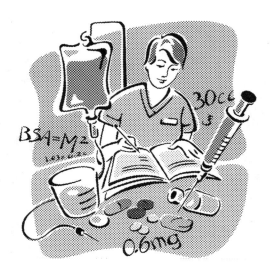

UNIT 2

Measurement Systems

Unit Objectives

Upon completion of this material, the learner will be able to:

- Identify metric, apothecary, and household equivalents.
- Solve metric problems by moving the decimal right or left.
- Convert Celsius and Fahrenheit temperatures.
- Convert from one unit of measurement to another:
  apothecary ⇌ household ⇌ metric ⇌ apothecary

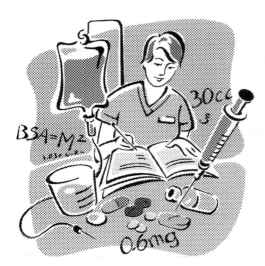

CHAPTER 5

Metric System

The **metric system** is an exact system of measurement in which units are expressed in multiples of 10. See Table 5.1.

Table 5.1
Metric Equivalents
The metric system of volume is based on the liter (1.06 qt).

Metric Volume
1 liter (L) = 1000 milliliters (ml)
1000 L = 1 kiloliter (kl)
1 ml = 1 cubic centimeter (cc)

The metric system of weight is based on the gram (g).
(453 g = 1 lb).

Metric Weight
1,000,000 micrograms (mcg) or (μg) = 1 gram (g)
1000 mcg = 1 milligram (mg)
1000 mg = 1 g
1000 g = 1 kilogram (kg) = 2.2 pounds (lb)

Metric Length
2.54 centimeters (cm) = 1 in

Because the units of the metric system are expressed in multiples of 10, problems can easily be solved by simply moving the decimal to the right or left (review rules for moving decimals in Chapter 2).

RULE

> When moving from large to small, move to the right ⟶
> and
> when moving from small to large, move to the left ⟵.
> One simple way to remember the rule:
>
> Large to small   (multiply)
> ⟶
> Small to large   (divide)
> ⟵

REMEMBER

> Metric answers are written in whole numbers and decimal fractions.

STEPS

> *To solve problems by moving the decimal*:
>
> 1. Determine which way to move the decimal—left or right.
>
> 2. Know the equivalent. Count the zeros in the equivalent.
>
> 3. Move the decimal the same number of places as there are zeros in the equivalent.

EXAMPLE:

$$45 \text{ g} = \underline{\hspace{1cm}} \text{ mcg}$$

1. $45 \text{ g} = \underline{\hspace{1cm}} \text{ mcg}$

      ↑   ↑
     Large **Small**

   To change large to small, ⟶ move the decimal to the right.
2. 1,000,000 mcg = 1 g—six zeros.
3. Move the decimal six places to the right:
   $$4\,5.000000. = 45,000,000$$

$$45 \text{ g} = 45,000,000 \text{ mcg}$$

EXAMPLE:

$$12 \text{ ml} = \underline{\hspace{1cm}} \text{ kl}$$

1. ml to kl is small to large. Move the decimal to the *left* ⟵.
2. We do not have an equivalent for ml to kl, but we do know that 1000 ml = 1 liter and 1000 L = 1 kl. So from ml to kl, there are six zeros, or six places.

3. Move the decimal to the left six places:

$$0.0000\overset{\curvearrowleft}{1}2 \ = \ 0.000012$$

12 ml   =   0.000012 kl

REMEMBER

When moving the decimal in the metric system, *do not round off the number.* All metric problems can also be solved by ratio and proportion—it just takes many steps, and the possibility for error is much greater. It is easy to make a mistake when dividing a number by 1,000,000. Learn to move the decimal. It is fast and easy.

PRACTICE PROBLEMS—MOVING THE DECIMAL

Move the decimal:

1. 529 mg = _____ g

2. 647 mcg = _____ mg

3. 42.7 g = _____ mcg

4. 804 mcg = _____ kg

5. 9.26 kg = _____ mg

6. 745 mg = _____ mcg

7. 85.4 mcg = _____ g

8. 5.28 kg = _____ g

9. 709 mg = _____ g

10. 34.3 g = _____ mg

11. 50.7 kg = _____ mcg

12. 238 g = _____ mcg

13. 7.93 kg = _____ mg

14. 75.4 mg = _____ g

15. 460 mcg = _____ kg

16. 659 kg = _____ g

17. 4.64 kg = _____ mg

18. 46.5 mg = _____ g

19. 743 g = _____ mcg

20. 529 mcg = _____ kg

21. 7.38 g = ____ kg

22. 23.4 kg = ____ mg

23. 387 mcg = ____ mg

24. 8.16 mg = ____ g

25. 3.3 mg = ____ g

26. 347 L = ____ ml

27. 1.35 kl = ____ cc

28. 851 ml = ____ kl

29. 729 ml = ____ cc

30. 52.1 kl = ____ ml

31. 41 cc = ____ L

32. 37 ml = ____ kl

33. 64.7 L = ____ cc

34. 83 kl = ____ ml

35. 26.5 ml = ____ cc

36. 69.52 ml = ____ kl

37. 48 L = ____ ml

38. 143 kl = ____ cc

39. 76 L = ____ kl

40. 93.2 cc = ____ kl

41. 115 kl = ____ ml

42. 84 ml = ____ kl

43. 4.24 L = ____ ml

44. 178 kl = ____ cc

45. 199 cc = ____ L

46. 29.42 kl = ____ L

47. 36.7 L = ____ cc

48. 3.97 ml = ____ kl

49. 296 ml = ____ L

50. 41.28 cc = ____ ml

51. 37.84 kg = ____ mg
= ____ mcg

52. 4.75 mg = ____ mcg

53. 219.6 mcg = _____ g
= _____ kg

54. 645 mg = _____ g

55. 28.3 g = _____ kg
= _____ mg

56. 6.03 g = _____ mcg

57. 4.564 mcg = _____ kg
= _____ g

58. 26.472 kg = _____ mg

59. 1.874 mg = _____ mcg
= _____ g

60. 876 g = _____ kg

61. 288 mcg = _____ mg
= _____ kg

62. 150 g = _____ mg

63. 83.56 kg = _____ mcg
= _____ mg

64. 57.429 g = _____ kg

65. 6.278 mcg = _____ g
= _____ mg

66. 209.5 mg = _____ g

67. 168 kg = _____ g

68. 417 mg = _____ mcg
= _____ g

69. 37.8 mg = _____ kg

70. 4.88 mcg = _____ mg
= _____ kg

71. 567 mg = _____ g

72. 5.84 kg = _____ mcg
= _____ mg

73. 225 mg = _____ kg

74. 3.36 kg = _____ mg
= _____ g

75. 238 mcg = _____ g

76. 439 ml = _____ cc
= _____ L

77. 7.53 kl = _____ L

78. 17.3 L = _____ cc
= _____ ml

79. 471 ml = _____ L

80. 3.28 ml = _____ kl
= _____ L

81. 238 kl = _____ cc

82. 59.4 L = _____ kl
= _____ cc

83. 199 ml = _____ L

84. 3.83 kl = _____ ml
    = _____ L

85. 3.94 ml = _____ L

86. 37 kl = _____ cc
    = _____ ml

87. 15.4 ml = _____ kl

88. 421 L = _____ cc
    = _____ kl

89. 239 cc = _____ L

90. 2.23 cc = _____ kl
    = _____ L

91. 28 ml = _____ L

92. 16.8 L = _____ kl
    = _____ cc

93. 103 ml = _____ cc

94. 10.1 kl = _____ ml
    = _____ L

95. 4.83 ml = _____ L

96. 26.7 cc = _____ kl
    = _____ ml

97. 198 L = _____ ml

98. 88 kl = _____ L
    = _____ cc

99. 35 ml = _____ cc

100. 4.26 cc = _____ kl
     = _____ L

Celsius and Fahrenheit

Celsius, the metric measurement of temperature, is used in most countries of the world. Sometimes the Celsius scale is called "centigrade" because the scale is divided into 100 parts. You are probably more familiar with the Fahrenheit scale. Both scales are based on the temperature of water.

FAHRENHEIT SCALE

212°	boiling point
32°	freezing point

CELSIUS SCALE

100°	boiling point
0°	freezing point

Thermometers used in hospitals in the United States measure temperature on a Fahrenheit or Celsius scale.

CHANGE CELSIUS TO FAHRENHEIT FORMULA

The formula for changing Celsius to Fahrenheit is:

$$°F = °C \times \frac{9}{5} + 32$$

EXAMPLE: A patient's temperature is 37° Celsius. Change to Fahrenheit.

$$°F = 37 \times \frac{9}{5} + 32$$
$$°F = \frac{333}{5} + 32$$
$$°F = 66.6 + 32$$
$$°F = \textbf{98.6}$$

CHANGE FAHRENHEIT TO CELSIUS FORMULA

The formula for changing Fahrenheit to Celsius is:

$$°C = \frac{5}{9} \times (°F - 32)$$

EXAMPLE: Today's outdoor temperature is 41°F. Change to Celsius.

$$°C = \frac{5}{9} \times (41 - 32)$$
$$°C = \frac{5}{9} \times 9$$
$$°C = \frac{5}{9} \times \frac{9}{1}$$
$$°C = \frac{45}{9}$$
$$°C = \textbf{5}$$

PRACTICE PROBLEMS—CELSIUS AND FAHRENHEIT

Solve:

1. 12°C = _____ °F

2. 49°C = _____°F

3. 69°C = _____ °F

4. 35°C = _____ °F

5. 72°C = _____ °F

6. 30°C = _____ °F

7. 107°C = _____ °F

8. 38°C = _____ °F

9. 59°C = _____ °F

10. 84°C = _____ °F

11. 80°F = _____ °C

16. 45°F = _____ °C

12. 100°F = _____ °C

17. 73°F = _____ °C

13. 32°F = _____ °C

18. 106°F = _____ °C

14. 59°F = _____ ° C

19. 90°F = _____ °C

15. 120°F = _____ °C

20. 102°F = _____ °C

ANSWERS

Moving the Decimal (pp. 59–62)

1. 0.529 g
2. 0.647 mg
3. 42,700,000 mcg
4. 0.000000804 kg
5. 9,260,000 mg
6. 745,000 mcg
7. 0.0000854 g
8. 5280 g
9. 0.709 g
10. 34,300 mg
11. 50,700,000,000 mcg
12. 238,000,000 mcg
13. 7,930,000 mg
14. 0.0754 g
15. 0.000000460 kg
16. 659,000 g
17. 4,640,000 mg
18. 0.0465 g
19. 743,000,000 mcg
20. 0.000000529 kg
21. 0.00738 kg
22. 23,400,000 mg
23. 0.387 mg
24. 0.00000816 kg
25. 0.0033 g
26. 346,000 ml

27. 1,350,000 cc
28. 0.000851 kl
29. 729 cc
30. 52,100,000 ml
31. 0.041 L
32. 0.000037 kl
33. 64,700 cc
34. 83,000,000 ml
35. 26.5 cc
36. 0.00006952 kl
37. 48,000 ml
38. 143,000,000 cc
39. 0.076 kl
40. 0.0000932 kl
41. 115,000,000 ml
42. 0.000084 kl
43. 4240 ml
44. 178,000,000 cc
45. 0.199 L
46. 29,420 L
47. 36,700 cc
48. 0.00000397 kl
49. 0.296 L
50. 41.28 ml
51. 37,840,000 mg
     37,840,000,000 mcg

52. 4750 mcg
53. 0.0002196 g
    0.0000002196 kg
54. 0.645 g
55. 0.0283 kg   28,300 mg
56. 6,030,000 mcg
57. 0.000000004564 kg
    0.000004564 g
58. 26,472,000 mg
59. 1874 mcg   0.001874 g
60. 0.876 kg
61. 0.288 mg   0.000000288 kg
62. 150,000 mg
63. 83,560,000,000 mcg
    83,560,000 mg
64. 0.057429 kg
65. 0.000006278 g
    0.006278 mg
66. 0.2095 g
67. 168,000 g
68. 417,000 mcg   0.417 g
69. 0.0000378 kg
70. 0.00488 mg   0.00000000488 kg
71. 0.567 g
72. 5,840,000,000 mcg
    5,840,000 mg
73. 0.000225 kg

74. 3,360,000 mg   3360 g
75. 0.000238 g
76. 439 cc   0.439 L
77. 7530 L
78. 17,300 cc   17,300 ml
79. 0.471 L
80. 0.00000328 kl   0.00328 L
81. 238,000,000 cc
82. 0.0594 kl   59,400 cc
83. 0.199 L
84. 3,830,000 ml   3830 L
85. 0.00394 L
86. 37,000,000 cc   37,000,000 ml
87. 0.0000154 kl
88. 421,000 cc   0.421 kl
89. 0.239 L
90. 0.00000223 kl   0.00223 L
91. 0.028 L
92. 0.0168 kl   16,800 cc
93. 103 cc
94. 10,100,000 ml   10,100 L
95. 0.00483 L
96. 0.0000267 kl   26.7 ml
97. 198,000 ml
98. 88,000 L   88,000,000 ml
99. 35 cc
100. 0.00000426 kl   0.00426 L

Celsius and Fahrenheit (pp. 63–64)

1. 53.6°F
2. 120.2°F
3. 156.2°F
4. 95°F
5. 161.6°F
6. 86°F
7. 224.6°F
8. 100.4°F
9. 138.2°F
10. 183.2°F
11. 26.67°C
12. 37.78°C
13. 0°C
14. 15°C
15. 48.89°C
16. 7.2°C
17. 22.78°C
18. 41.1°C
19. 32.2°C
20. 38.89°C

CHAPTER 6

Apothecary and Household Measurements

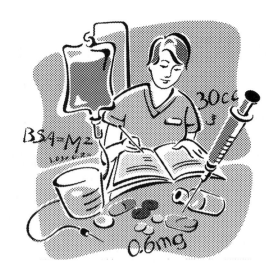

Although most drugs are ordered in the metric unit of measurement, some physicians and advanced practice nurses may use the apothecary unit. Household measurements are occasionally used when instructing proper dosage to take at home.

Apothecary symbols may precede or follow the amount. The number may be expressed in Arabic numerals or in Roman numerals. For example, 24 ℨ and ℨ xxiv are equal expressions.

It is necessary to learn the following equivalents in Table 6.1. ≃ is the symbol used to designate approximate equivalents.

REMEMBER	The apothecary system will not be as exact as the metric system.

Table 6.1
Household and Apothecary Equivalents

Household		Apothecary
		Weight
		60 gr (grains) = 1 ℨ (dram)
		8 ℨ = 1 ℥ (oz)
	Liquid	
15–16 gtt (drops)	≃	15–16 m_x (minim)
1 tsp	≃	1 ℨ
1 Tbsp	≃	4 ℨ ≃ $\frac{1}{2}$ ℥
2 Tbsp	≃	8 ℨ = ℥
1 teacup	=	6 ℥
1 glass	=	8 ℥
1 pt	=	16 ℥
2 pt = 1 qt	=	32 ℥
4 qt = 1 gal	=	128 ℥

FIGURE 6.1 Medication cup showing apothecary and household measurements.

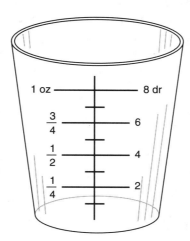 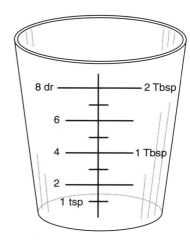

To solve apothecary and household problems, use the principles of *ratio and proportion*. Begin each problem with the known equivalent and then solve for X. In working problems in this system, you can use either value when a range is given.

REMEMBER

For consistency in working problems, the authors have elected to always use the larger number in the equivalent range.

RULE

In the apothecary unit of measurement, numerical fractions are used to express less than whole numbers.

STEPS

1. Write known equivalent.

2. Identify unknown factor and known factor.

3. Cross-multiply to solve for X.

EXAMPLE: How many ℥ are in 16 ℥?

Known equivalent: $\frac{8℥}{1℥} = \frac{X}{16℥}$

Cross-multiply to solve for X.

$$X = 8 \times 16$$
$$X = \textbf{128 ℥}$$

EXAMPLE: 6 ℥ = _____ ℥ = _____ glass.

(a) $\frac{8℥}{1℥} = \frac{6℥}{X}$

$$8X = 6$$
$$X = \frac{6}{8} = \frac{3}{4}$$
$$X = \frac{3}{4}℥$$

(b) $\frac{8℥}{1 \text{ glass}} = \frac{\frac{3}{4}℥}{X}$

$$8X = \frac{3}{4}$$
$$X = \frac{3}{4} \times \frac{1}{8}$$
$$X = \frac{3}{32} \textbf{ glass}$$

PRACTICE PROBLEMS—APOTHECARY AND HOUSEHOLD PROBLEMS

Solve:

1. 4 tsp = _____ ʒ

2. ʒ $\overline{X}$ = _____ tsp

3. 4 pt = _____ qt

4. 25 tsp = _____ ʒ

5. 180 gr = _____ ʒ

6. ʒ $\overline{xxiv}$ = _____ ʒ

7. 24 ʒ = _____ glasses = _____ pt

8. 3 tsp = _____ ʒ

9. 80 tsp = _____ ʒ = _____ ʒ

10. 6 qt = _____ pt

11. 4 tsp = _____ ʒ

12. ʒ $\overline{xii}$ = _____ teacups

13. 20 ʒ = _____ gr = _____ ʒ

14. ʒ $\overline{xiv}$ = _____ ʒ

15. 3$\frac{1}{2}$ teacups = _____ ʒ

16. $\frac{3}{4}$ ʒ = _____ ʒ

17. 5 glasses = _____ ʒ = _____ pt

18. 75 gtt = _____ m_x

19. 2 gal = _____ qt = _____ pt

20. $\frac{1}{2}$ Tbsp = _____ ʒ

21. 6 pt = _____ ʒ = _____ qt

22. 5 ʒ = _____ ʒ

23. 2$\frac{1}{2}$ qt = _____ gal = _____ ʒ

24. ʒ $\overline{ss}$ = _____ tsp

25. 1080 gtt = _____ m_x

26. The order reads Benylin cough syrup $\frac{1}{4}$ ℥. How many 3 will that be?

27. A mother is told to give her child 2 3 of medication four times a day. How many teaspoons should she give the child each time?

28. How many gr are in 4 3?

29. If you had to measure 2 gal of water and only had a pt container, how many pt would you use?

30. A patient is told to drink 48 oz of fluid every day. You advise the patient to drink how many teacups full per day?

31. In measuring 3 $\overline{\text{xv}}$ of a liquid, you would have how many ℥?

32: In giving 6 tsp of a medication, you could use how many 3?

33. If your patient drank a pint of juice, how many oz would he have consumed?

34. Change ℥ $\overline{\overline{\text{xxx}}}$ to 3.

35. To give 3 $\overline{\text{V}}$, you advise the mother to use how many tsp?

36. How many ℥ are in 2 qt?

37. Your patient drank ℥ $\overline{\text{vi}}$ of juice and ℥ $\overline{\overline{\text{iii}}}$ of water. How many ℥ did he drink?

38. If a patient drank 14 glasses of liquid a day, how many ℥ would that equal?

39. For your patient to drink a total of 64 ℥ per day, you would have the patient drink how many glasses?

40. To give ℥ $\overline{\text{xxv}}$, you would measure how many Tbsp?

41. To give $\frac{3}{4}$ ℥, you would measure how many ʒ?

42. How many ℥ are in 14 ʒ?

43. A patient had 2 pt of juice. How many ℥ did he have?

44. In giving ℥ $\overline{\text{iss}}$, you will have how many ʒ?

45. In order to insure that your patient drinks ℥ $\overline{\text{xxx}}$ during your shift, you need to have him drink how many glasses?

46. A patient whose liquid intake is limited to 50 oz per day should drink how many glasses of liquid?

47. How many qt are in 4 gal?

48. To give $\frac{3}{4}$ Tbsp, you would measure how many tsp?

49. An order reads Penicillin ℥ xii. You know this will be how many ʒ?

50. If your patient drank $2\frac{1}{2}$ pt of liquid over an eight hour period, how many ʒ would this be?

ANSWERS

Apothecary and Household Problems (pp. 68–71)

1. $\frac{1}{2}$ ʒ	18. 75 m_x	35. 5 tsp
2. 10 tsp	19. 8 qt, 16 pt	36. 64 ʒ
3. 2 qt	20. 2 ʒ	37. $1\frac{1}{8}$ ʒ
4. 25 ʒ	21. 96 ʒ, 3 qts	38. 112 ʒ
5. 3 ʒ	22. $\frac{5}{8}$ ʒ	39. 8 glasses
6. 3 ʒ	23. $\frac{5}{8}$ gal, 80 ʒ	40. $6\frac{1}{4}$ Tbsp
7. 3 glasses, $1\frac{1}{2}$ pt	24. 4 tsp	41. 6 ʒ
8. $\frac{3}{8}$ ʒ or $\frac{1}{2}$ oz	25. 1080 m_x	42. $1\frac{3}{4}$ ʒ
9. 80 ʒ, 10 ʒ	26. 2 ʒ	43. 32 ʒ
10. 12 pt	27. 2 tsp	44. 12 ʒ
11. 4 ʒ	28. 240 gr	45. $3\frac{3}{4}$ ʒ
12. 2 teacups	29. 16 pt	46. $6\frac{1}{4}$ glasses
13. 1200 gr, $2\frac{1}{2}$ ʒ	30. 8 teacups	47. 16 qt
14. $1\frac{3}{4}$ ʒ	31. $1\frac{7}{8}$ ʒ	48. 3 tsp
15. 21 ʒ	32. 6 ʒ	49. $1\frac{1}{2}$ ʒ
16. 6 ʒ	33. 16 ʒ	50. 40 ʒ
17. 40 ʒ, $2\frac{1}{2}$ pt	34. 240 ʒ	

CHAPTER 7

Metric, Apothecary, and Household Conversions

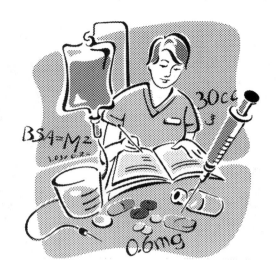

Medications may be ordered in Metric, Apothecary or Household units. In order to give medications, the nurse must be able to convert from one system to another. After studying the equivalents on Table 7.1 and using the previously learned material, the learner should be able to convert from each system successfully.

Table 7.1 *Equivalents*		
Household	Apothecary	Metric
	Weight	
	1 gr =	60 mg
	60 gr = 1 ʒ (dram)	
	8 ʒ = 1 ℥ (oz)	
	Liquid	
15–16 gtt (drops)	≃ 15–16 m_x (minim)	1 ml (cc)
1 tsp	≃ 1 ʒ	4–5 ml
1 Tbsp	≃ 4 ʒ	15–16 ml
2 Tbsp	≃ 8 ʒ = 1 ℥	30 ml
1 teacup	= 6 ℥	180 ml
1 glass	= 8 ℥	240 ml
1 pt	= 16 ℥	500 ml
2 pt = 1 qt	= 32 ℥	1000 ml = 1 Liter (L)
4 qt = 1 gal	= 128 ℥	

To convert one measurement system to another, use ratio-proportion principles. Each problem must begin with the known equivalent.

EXAMPLE: To change $\frac{1}{4}$ gr to mg, you must know that 60 mg = 1 gr.

Known equivalent: $\dfrac{60 \text{ mg}}{1 \text{ gr}} = \dfrac{X \text{ mg}}{\frac{1}{4} \text{ gr}}$

Cross-multiply to solve for X.

$$X = 60 \times \tfrac{1}{4}$$
$$X = \tfrac{60}{4}$$
$$X = \textbf{15 mg}$$

FIGURE 7.1 Medication cup showing apothecary and metric measurements.

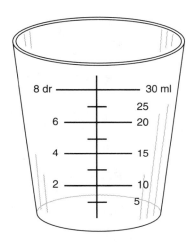

EXAMPLE: Change 10 mg to gr.

Known equivalent: $\dfrac{60 \text{ mg}}{1 \text{ gr}} = \dfrac{10 \text{ mg}}{X \text{ gr}}$

$$60 X = 10$$
$$X = \tfrac{10}{60}$$
$$X = \tfrac{1}{6} \textbf{ gr}$$

Approximate Equivalents

When converting between the metric and apothecary systems of measurement, we usually use the equivalent 60 mg = 1 gr. There are times, however, when approximate equivalents appear in problems. In these instances, do not compute the answer using 60 mg = 1 gr. Just recognize the approximate equivalent, as seen in Table 7.2, and write the appropriate answer.

Table 7.2
Approximate Equivalents

$50 \text{ mg} \simeq \frac{3}{4} \text{ gr}$	$300\text{--}325 \text{ mg} \simeq 5 \text{ gr}$
$100 \text{ mg} \simeq 1\frac{1}{2} \text{ gr}$	$500 \text{ mg} \simeq 7\frac{1}{2} \text{ gr}$
$200 \text{ mg} \simeq 3 \text{ gr}$	$1000 \text{ mg} \simeq 15 \text{ gr}$
$250 \text{ mg} \simeq 3\frac{3}{4} \text{ gr}$	

EXAMPLE: The order is written to give Seconal $1\frac{1}{2}$ gr. How many milligrams is this?

100 mg

If the problem had been worked with 60 mg = 1 gr, the answer derived would have been 90. That is incorrect.

EXAMPLE: Give 50 mg of Demerol. How many grains is this?

$\frac{3}{4}$ *gr*

You must know the approximate equivalent table as well as the other measurement tables.

PRACTICE PROBLEMS—APPROXIMATE EQUIVALENTS

Solve:

1. 15 gr = _____ mg

2. 19 ml = _____ m_x

3. 0.25 g = _____ gr
   = _____ mg

4. 15 mg = _____ gr

5. $\frac{1}{8}$ gr = _____ mg

6. 39 kg = _____ lb

7. ℥ iv = _____ tsp

8. 15 ml = _____ ℥

9. $\frac{1}{2}$ gal = _____ ml
   = _____ qt

10. 250 ml = _____ pt

11. 16 ml = _____ ℥
    = _____ Tbsp

12. 750 mg = _____ gr

13. 750 ml = _____ qt

26. 0.1 mg = _____ gr

14. 3 g = _____ gr
       = _____ mg

27. 15 ml = _____ ʒ

15. $\frac{1}{150}$ gr = _____ mg

28. $\frac{1}{60}$ gr = _____ mg
       = _____ g

16. 0.6 mg = _____ gr
       = _____ g

29. 60 ml = _____ Tbsp

17. 400 g = _____ mg
       = _____ gr

30. 4 teacups = _____ ml

18. $\frac{1}{200}$ gr = _____ mg

31. 360 ml = _____ glasses

19. ʒ $\overline{ss}$ = _____ ml

32. 16 ʒ = _____ ml

20. 60 ml = _____ tsp

33. $\frac{1}{600}$ gr = _____ mg
       = _____ g

21. 64 ʒ = _____ L

34. 3500 ml = _____ pt

22. 45 ml = _____ ʒ

35. 2.5 L = _____ qt

23. 79 kg = _____ lb

36. 6 qt = _____ ml

24. 250 mg = _____ gr

37. 150 mg = _____ gr

25. 12 ml = _____ gtt

38. 10 kg = _____ lb

39. 75 cc = _____ m$_x$

40. ℥ $\overline{\text{xvi}}$ = _____ ʒ

41. 10 mg = _____ gr

42. 120 cc = _____ ʒ

43. 3 ʒ = _____ ml

44. gr $\overline{\text{iss}}$ = _____ mg
        = _____ g

45. 1500 ml = _____ pt

46. 250 mg = _____ gr

47. 4728 cc = _____ qt
         = _____ L

48. 0.15 ml = _____ gtt

49. 1.5 g = _____ mg
    = _____ gr

50. 500 mg = _____ gr

51. 110 kg = _____ lb
     = _____ g

52. $\frac{3}{4}$ gr = _____ mg

53. 0.3 g = _____ mg
     = _____ gr

54. 100 ml = _____ gtt

55. 380 cc = _____ ʒ
      = _____ ℥

56. 150 ml = _____ ℥

57. 2 Tbsp = _____ ml

58. 7 pt = _____ qt

59. $\frac{1}{400}$ gr = _____ mg

60. 300 cc = _____ pt
      = _____ qt

61. 0.3 mg = _____ gr
      = _____ g

62. 2750 cc = _____ qt

63. $\frac{1}{4}$ gr = _____ mg

64. 12 mg = _____ gr

65. $\overline{3}\,\overline{xv}$ = _____ ml

78. 25 kg = _____ lb

66. 800 mg = _____ gr

79. 225 ml = _____ gtt

67. $\frac{1}{100}$ gr = _____ mg

80. 710 cc = _____ $\overline{3}$
     = _____ L

68. 95 kg = _____ lb

81. 492 ml = _____ $\overline{3}$

69. gr $\overline{viiss}$ = _____ mg
     = _____ g

82. 100 ml = _____ tsp

70. 978 ml = _____ 3

83. 75 ml = _____ Tbsp

71. 27 cc = _____ m_x
     = _____ tsp

84. 2 kg = _____ mg

72. 120 cc = _____ tsp

85. 50 mg = _____ gr

73. 450 cc = _____ Tbsp
     = _____ 3

86. 160.02 cm = _____ in

74. 10 L = _____ pt

87. 198.12 cm = _____ in

75. 1000 ml = _____ gal
      = _____ pt

88. 162.56 cm = _____ in

76. 0.75 kg = _____ gr

89. 182.88 cm = _____ in

77. 300 mg = _____ gr
     = _____ g

90. 152.4 cm = _____ in

ANSWERS

Approximate Equivalents (pp. 74–77)

1. 1000 mg
2. 304 m_x
3. $3\frac{3}{4}$ gr, 250 mg
4. $\frac{1}{4}$ gr
5. 7.5 mg
6. 85.8 lb
7. 4 tsp
8. $\frac{1}{2}$ ʒ
9. 2000 ml, 2 qt
10. $\frac{1}{2}$ pt
11. 4 ʒ, 1 Tbsp
12. $12\frac{1}{2}$ gr
13. $\frac{3}{4}$ qt
14. 50 gr, 3000 mg
15. 0.4 mg
16. $\frac{1}{100}$ gr, 0.0006 g
17. 400,000 mg, 6000, or $6666\frac{2}{3}$ gr
18. 0.3 mg
19. 15 ml
20. 12 tsp
21. 2 L
22. 9 ʒ
23. 173.8 lb
24. $3\frac{3}{4}$ gr
25. 192 gtt
26. $\frac{1}{600}$ gr
27. 3 ʒ
28. 1 mg, 0.001 g
29. $3\frac{3}{4}$ Tbsp
30. 720 ml
31. $1\frac{1}{2}$ glasses
32. 500 ml
33. 0.1 mg, 0.0001 g
34. 7 pt
35. $2\frac{1}{2}$ qt
36. 6000 ml
37. $2\frac{1}{2}$ gr
38. 22 lb
39. 1200 m_x
40. 2 ʒ
41. $\frac{1}{6}$ gr
42. 24 ʒ
43. 90 ml
44. 100 mg, 0.1 g
45. 3 pt
46. $3\frac{3}{4}$ gr
47. $4\frac{91}{125}$ qt, 4.728 L
48. $2\frac{2}{5}$ gtt
49. 1500 mg, 25 gr
50. $7\frac{1}{2}$ gr

51. 242 lb, 110,000 g

52. 50 mg

53. 300 mg, 5 gr

54. 1600 gtt

55. 76 ℥, $9\frac{1}{2}$ ℥ or $12\frac{2}{3}$ ℥

56. 5 ℥

57. 32 ml

58. $3\frac{1}{2}$ qt

59. 0.15 mg

60. $\frac{3}{5}$ pt, $\frac{3}{10}$ qt

61. $\frac{1}{200}$ gr, 0.0003 g

62. $2\frac{3}{4}$ qt

63. 15 mg

64. $\frac{1}{5}$ gr

65. 75 ml

66. $13\frac{1}{3}$ gr

67. 0.6 mg

68. 209 lb

69. 500 mg, 0.5 g

70. $195\frac{3}{5}$ ℥

71. 432 m_x, $5\frac{2}{5}$ tsp

72. 24 tsp

73. $28\frac{1}{8}$ Tbsp, 90 ℥

74. 20 pt

75. $\frac{1}{4}$ gal, 2 pt

76. 11,250 gr

77. 5 gr, 0.3 g

78. 55 lb

79. 3600 gtt

80. 142 ℥, 0.71 L

81. $16\frac{2}{5}$ ℥

82. 20 tsp

83. $4\frac{11}{16}$ Tbsp

84. 2,000,000 mg

85. $\frac{3}{4}$ gr

86. 63 in

87. 78 in

88. 64 in

89. 72 in

90. 60 in

UNIT 2

Comprehensive Test

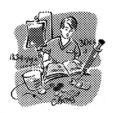

Calculate the following metric, apothecary, and household problems:

1. 216 ml = _____ L
   = _____ cc

2. 804 L = _____ kl

3. 250 cc = _____ ml
   = _____ L

4. 4854 ml = _____ kl

5. 6.328 kl = _____ L
   = _____ ml

6. 21.60 ml = _____ L

7. 340 L = _____ cc
   = _____ kl

8. 242.4 kl = _____ cc

9. 1755 cc = _____ L
   = _____ ml

10. 310.7 L = _____ kl

11. 4240 cc = _____ kl
    = _____ L

12. 45.63 ml = _____ cc

13. 510 kl = _____ ml
    = _____ L

14. 1320 L = _____ ml

15. 21,014 cc = _____ kl
    = _____ ml

16. 90,009 L = _____ kl

17. 4816 ml = _____ L
    = _____ cc

30. 2 tsp = _____ ml

18. 5212 mcg = _____ g

31. 16 ʒ = _____ ml

19. 14,000 mcg = _____ mg
    = _____ g

32. 20 gr = _____ ʒ

20. 1248 mg = _____ g

33. 3 pt = _____ ʒ
    = _____ ml

21. 2807 kg = _____ g
    = _____ mg

34. 26 ʒ = _____ glasses

22. 5664 g = _____ kg

35. 32 m_x = _____ ml
    = _____ gtt

23. 29,700 g = _____ mg
    = _____ mcg

36. 60 ml = _____ ʒ

24. 378 mg = _____ mcg

37. 5 Tbsp = _____ ml

25. 652 g = _____ mcg
    = _____ kg

38. 360 ml = _____ ʒ

26. 100 ml = _____ ʒ

39. 64 ʒ = _____ ml
    = _____ pt

27. 6 qt = _____ gal
    = _____ pt

40. 3 glasses = _____ ml

28. 4 glasses = _____ ml

41. 16 ml = _____ m_x

29. 15 ml = _____ ʒ
    = _____ ʒ

42. 120 m_x = _____ ml

43. $2\frac{1}{2}$ qt = _____ ℥
    = _____ ml

44. 45 ml = _____ tsp

45. 750 ml = _____ pt
    = _____ ℥

46. 847 mcg = _____ g

47. 6.52 mg = _____ mcg
    = _____ g

48. 847 mg = _____ g

49. 6378 g = _____ kg
    = _____ mg

50. 9856 mg = _____ kg

51. 568 kg = _____ g
    = _____ mg

52. 78.4 g = _____ mg

53. 79°F = _____ °C

54. 68°C = _____ °F

55. 30 cc = _____ gtt
    = _____ ml

56. 10.16 cm = _____ in

57. 480 ml = _____ ℥

58. 24 ml = _____ ℨ

59. 500 mg = _____ gr
    = _____ g

60. 1750 ml = _____ qt

61. 2 gal = _____ ml
    = _____ qt

62. 4 ℨ = _____ glass

63. $\frac{1}{6}$ gr = _____ mg
    = _____ g

64. 8 Tbsp = _____ ℨ

65. 5 pt = _____ ℥
    = _____ ml

66. ℨ $\overline{\text{vi}}$ = _____ ml

67. 7 qt = _____ pt

68. 3 teacups = _____ ℥

69. 8 glasses = _____ ml

70. 90 m_x = _____ ℨ

71. 4 pt = _____ ℨ
= _____ ml

72. ℨ $\overline{\overline{iii}}$ = _____ ml

73. $\frac{1}{300}$ gr = _____ mg
= _____ g

74. ℨ $\overline{viii}$ = _____ ml

75. 1 gal = _____ ℨ
= _____ ml

76. 6 teacups = _____ ℨ

77. 20 ℨ = _____ ℨ

78. 16 Tbsp = _____ ml

79. 5 gr = _____ mg
= _____ g

80. 8 pt = _____ ml

81. ℨ $\overline{\overline{iiss}}$ = _____ ml

82. 30 gr = _____ ℨ

83. 6 glasses = _____ ml

84. 180 m_x = _____ tsp

85. 3 gr = _____ mg
= _____ g

86. $\frac{1}{250}$ gr = _____ mg

87. 10 ℨ = _____ ml

88. $2\frac{1}{2}$ teacups = _____ ml

89. 3 qt = _____ ml

90. $\frac{1}{3}$ gr = _____ mg

91. ℨ $\overline{iv}$ = _____ ml

92. 241.3 cm = _____ in

93. 0.4 mg = _____ gr
= _____ g

94. 30 kg = _____ lb

95. 0.5 ml = _____ gtt = _____ L   **98.** 15 ml = _____ ℥

96. 0.2 mg = _____ gr   **99.** 0.1 mg = _____ gr
                                             = _____ g

97. 0.25 L = _____ ℥   **100.** $2\frac{1}{2}$ cc = _____ m_x
             = _____ ℨ

ANSWERS

Unit 2: Comprehensive Test (pp. 80–84)

1. 0.216 L, 216 cc		**19.** 14 mg, 0.014 g
2. 0.804 kl		**20.** 1.248 g
3. 250 ml, 0.25 L		**21.** 2,807,000 g,
4. 0.004854 kl		2,807,000,000 mg
5. 6328 L, 6,328,000 ml		**22.** 5.664 kg
6. 0.0216 L		**23.** 29,700,000 mg
7. 340,000 cc, 0.34 kl		29,700,000,000 mcg
8. 242,400,000 cc		**24.** 378,000 mcg
9. 1.755 L, 1755 ml		**25.** 652,000,000 mcg, 0.652 kg
10. 0.3107 kl		**26.** $3\frac{1}{3}$ ℥
11. 0.00424 kl, 4.24 L		**27.** $1\frac{1}{2}$ gal, 12 pt
12. 45.63 cc		**28.** 960 ml
13. 510,000,000 ml, 510,000 L		**29.** 4 ℥, $\frac{1}{2}$ ℥
14. 1,320,000 ml		**30.** 10 ml
15. 0.021014 kl, 21,014 ml		**31.** 80 ml
16. 90.009 kl		**32.** $\frac{1}{3}$ ℥
17. 4.816 L, 4816 cc		**33.** 48 ℥, 1500 ml
18. 0.005212 g		**34.** $3\frac{1}{4}$ glasses

35. 2 ml, 32 gtt

36. 2 ʒ

37. 80 ml

38. 12 ʒ

39. 1920 ml, 4 pt

40. 720 ml

41. 256 m_x

42. 7.5 ml

43. 80 ʒ, 2500 ml

44. 9 tsp

45. $1\frac{1}{2}$ pt, 24 or 25 ʒ

46. 0.000847 g

47. 6520 mcg, 0.00652 g

48. 0.847 g

49. 6.378 kg, 6,378,000 mg

50. 0.009856 kg

51. 568,000 g, 568,000,000 mg

52. 78,400 mg

53. 26.1°C

54. 154.4°F

55. 480 gtt, 30 ml

56. 4 in

57. 16 ʒ

58. $4\frac{4}{5}$ ʒ

59. $7\frac{1}{2}$ gr, 0.5 g

60. $1\frac{3}{4}$ qt

61. 8000 ml, 8 qt

62. $\frac{1}{2}$ glass

63. 10 mg, 0.01 g

64. 32 ʒ

65. 80 ʒ, 2500 ml

66. 30 ml

67. 14 pt

68. 18 ʒ

69. 1920 ml

70. $1\frac{1}{8}$ ʒ

71. 64 ʒ, 2000 ml

72. 15 ml

73. 0.2 mg, 0.0002 g

74. 240 ml

75. 128 ʒ, 4000 ml

76. 36 ʒ

77. $2\frac{1}{2}$ ʒ

78. 256 ml

79. 300 mg, 0.3 g

80. 4000 ml

81. 75 ml

82. $\frac{1}{2}$ ʒ

83. 1440 ml

84. $2\frac{1}{4}$ tsp

85. 200 mg, 0.2 g

86. 0.24 mg

87. 50 ml

88. 450 ml

89. 3000 ml

90. 20 mg

91. 120 ml

92. 95 in

93. $\frac{1}{150}$ gr, 0.0004 g

94. 66 lb

95. 8 gtt, 0.0005 L

96. $\frac{1}{300}$ gr

97. 8 ℥, 64 ʒ

98. $\frac{1}{2}$ ʒ

99. $\frac{1}{600}$ gr, 0.0001 g

100. 40 m_x

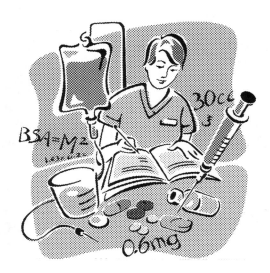

UNIT 3

Drugs and Solutions

Unit Objectives

Upon completion of this material, the learner will be able to:

- Convert traditional time to Universal (military) time and Universal (military) time to traditional time.
- Solve oral dosage problems involving tablets, liquids, and capsules using the formula $\frac{D}{H} \times$ Amount.
- Solve parenteral dosage problems using drugs in solution and in powdered form.
- Calculate IV drip rates using various administration sets.
- Calculate titrated drug dosages.
- Solve children's dosage problems using BSA, kg of body weight, and traditional rules.

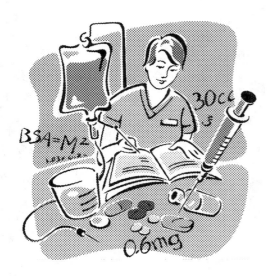

CHAPTER 8

Medication Administration

How to Use Universal (Military) Time

Many health care facilities use Universal time instead of A.M. and P.M. time, in order to avoid confusion and clarify documentation. Figures 8.1 and 8.2 show the relationship between traditional and universal times.

Universal time is based on a 24-hour clock, which begins at 0001 or one minute after midnight. 1 A.M. is 0100. After noon, add 1200 to the hour. Example: 3 P.M. is 3 + 1200 = 1500.

FIGURE 8.1 A.M. Clock

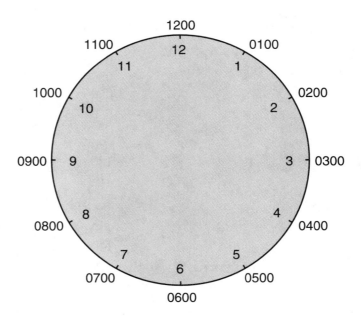

FIGURE 8.2 P.M. Clock

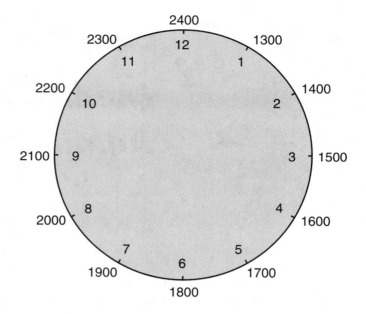

Table 8.1	
Time Table	
Universal Time	Traditional Time
0030	30 minutes past midnight
0100	1:00 A.M.
0130	1:30 A.M.
0200	2:00 A.M.
0300	3:00 A.M.
0400	4:00 A.M.
0500	5:00 A.M.
0600	6:00 A.M.
0700	7:00 A.M.
0800	8:00 A.M.
0900	9:00 A.M.
1000	10:00 A.M.
1100	11:00 A.M.
1200	12:00 P.M. noon
1230	12:30 P.M.
1300	1:00 P.M.
1400	2:00 P.M.
1500	3:00 P.M.
1600	4:00 P.M.
1700	5:00 P.M.
1800	6:00 P.M.
1900	7:00 P.M.
2000	8:00 P.M.
2100	9:00 P.M.
2200	10:00 P.M.
2300	11:00 P.M.
2400	12:00 A.M. midnight

How to Set Up Medication Schedules

There are some commonly used abbreviations for medication schedules. These abbreviations are used in health care facilities and in prescribing medications. When used in a health care facility, the schedule may vary with the institution. A nurse should always become familiar with the hours designated by a specific institution.

Table 8.2 shows some examples of commonly used abbreviations and time schedules.

Table 8.2 *Suggested Time Schedule*		
	Traditional	Universal
qd = every day	9 A.M.	0900
qod = every other day	9 A.M. alt. days	0900 alt. days
bid = twice a day	9 A.M., 5 P.M.	0900, 1700
tid = three times a day	9 A.M., 1 P.M., 5 P.M.	0900, 1300, 1700
qid = four times a day	9 A.M., 1 P.M., 5 P.M., 9 P.M.	0900, 1300, 1700, 2100
q4h = every four hours	9 A.M., 1 P.M., 5 P.M., 9 P.M., 1 A.M., 5 A.M.	0900, 1300, 1700, 2100, 0100, 0500
q6h = every six hours	12 midnight, 6 A.M., 12 noon, 6 P.M.	2400, 0600, 1200, 1800
q8h = every eight hours	6 A.M., 2 P.M., 10 P.M.	0600, 1400, 2200
H.S. or hs = hour of sleep (bedtime)	9 P.M.	2100
AC = before meals	7:30 A.M., 11:30 A.M., 4:30 P.M.	0730, 1130, 1630
PC = after meals	9 A.M., 1 P.M., 6 P.M.	0900, 1300, 1800

How to Interpret Abbreviations

Abbreviations are used in many areas of nursing. Table 8.3 contains a sample of some of the most common abbreviations. Each institution has an accepted list of abbreviations. The nurse should only use those abbreviations that have been approved by the employing facility.

Table 8.3 *Abbreviations*					
po	=	by mouth (per os)	oint	=	ointment
SL or sub ling	=	sublinguinal (under tongue)	KVO	=	keep vein open
supp	=	suppository	STAT	=	immediately
susp	=	suspension	$\bar{c}$	=	with
tr	=	tincture	$\bar{S}$	=	without
IM	=	intramuscular	PRN	=	when needed
SQ, SC or Sub q	=	subcutaneous	OD	=	right eye
IV	=	intravenous	OS	=	left eye
IVPB	=	intravenous piggyback	OU	=	both eyes
IVP	=	intravenous push	AC	=	before meals
pr	=	per rectal	PC	=	after meals
IVf	=	intravenous fluid	h.s.	=	at bedtime (hour of sleep)

How to Read a Drug Label

Always read each label carefully. Look for both the generic and trademark names. The generic name comes from one of three sources: 1) the biochemical name, 2) the name assigned by the U.S. Adopted Names Council, or 3) the name given since antiquity. The trademark name (trade name, proprietary name) is the name given to the drug by the manufacturer. This is a registered name, and the symbol ® is always found at the upper-right of the trademark name.

There is other important information on the label. Look for the amount of medication contained in the tablet, liquid, ampule, vial, etc. The route of administration may be given. If the drug is in powder form, directions for dilution are usually on the vial label, or the label will state, "Refer to package insert for reconstitution." Also included are the name of the manufacturer and the total amount of drug in the ampule or vial, as seen in Figure 8.3.

FIGURE 8.3

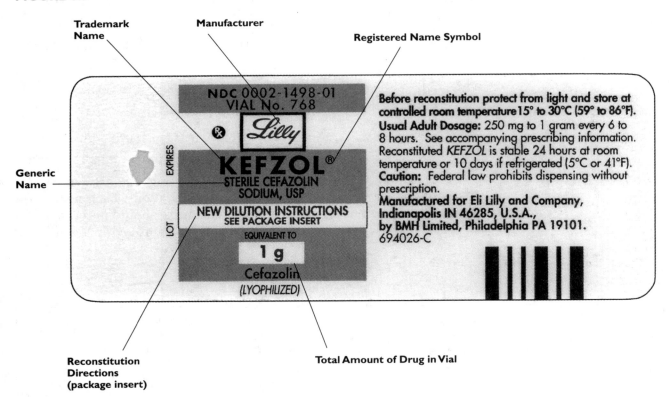

Used with permission from Eli Lilly and Company, Inc.

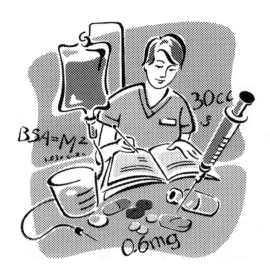

CHAPTER 9

Oral Medications

Oral medications usually come in the dosage ordered. There are times, however, when the nurse must calculate the number or portion of tablets or the amount of liquid to administer. The first step in solving these problems is to make sure the desired dosage (D) and the dosage on hand (H) are in the same units of measurement.

STEPS

1. Convert to the same unit of measurement if necessary.

2. Use the formula: $\dfrac{\text{D (Desired dose)}}{\text{H (Dosage on hand)}} = \text{Amount to give}$

3. Or if medication is in liquid form, use:

$$\dfrac{\text{D (Desired dose)}}{\text{H (Dosage on hand)}} \times \begin{array}{c}\text{Amount}\\\text{of liquid}\end{array} = \text{Amount to give}$$

EXAMPLE: To administer $\frac{1}{8}$ gr of a drug which is available in 15 mg tablets, you must convert $\frac{1}{8}$ gr to mg, or 15 mg to gr.

(a) $\dfrac{60 \text{ mg}}{1 \text{ gr}} = \dfrac{X \text{ mg}}{\frac{1}{8} \text{ gr}}$

$X = 60 \times \frac{1}{8}$

$X = \frac{60}{8}$

$X = \textbf{7.5 mg}$

(b) $\dfrac{60 \text{ mg}}{1 \text{ gr}} = \dfrac{15 \text{ mg}}{X \text{ gr}}$

$60X = 15$

$X = \frac{15}{60}$

$X = \frac{1}{4} \textbf{ gr}$

The next step is to use the formula.

$$\frac{D}{H} = \text{Amount to give} \qquad \frac{\text{Dosage desired}}{\text{Dosage on hand}} = \text{Amount to give}$$

$$\frac{\frac{1}{8}\,\text{gr}}{\frac{1}{4}\,\text{gr}} = \frac{4}{8} = \frac{1}{2}\,\textbf{tablet} \quad \text{or} \quad \frac{7.5\,\text{mg}}{15\,\text{mg}} = \frac{1}{2}\,\textbf{tablet}$$

REMEMBER

It is possible to give part of a scored tablet; however, it is not possible to give part of a capsule.

EXAMPLE: Give 4 mg of a drug that comes in 2 mg tablets.

$$\frac{\text{Desired dosage}}{\text{Dosage on hand}} = \frac{4\,\text{mg}}{2\,\text{mg}} = \textbf{2 tablets}$$

RULE

Liquid Form
To give a drug which comes in a liquid form, the formula to use is:
$$\frac{D}{H} \times \text{Amount of liquid} = \text{Amount to give}$$

EXAMPLE: Give 125 mg of a liquid medication which comes as 250 mg per 5 ml.

$$\frac{125}{250} \times 5$$

$$\frac{1}{2} \times 5 = \textbf{2.5 ml}$$

REMEMBER

Step 1: **Convert the measurement system if necessary.**
Step 2: **Use the formula to solve for drug dosage.**

$$\frac{\text{Desired dosage}}{\text{Dose on hand}} = \text{Amount to give}$$

$$\frac{\text{Desired dosage}}{\text{Dose on hand}} \times \text{Amount of liquid} = \text{Amount to give}$$

PRACTICE PROBLEMS — ORAL MEDICATIONS

Solve:

1. Ordered: Amoxicillin 0.25 g po q6h
   On hand: Amoxicillin 125 mg capsule   Give _____ cap

2. Ordered: Albuterol 6 mg po tid
   On hand: Albuterol 2 mg tablet   Give _____ tab

3. Ordered: Captopril 50 mg po tid
   On hand: Captopril 12.5 mg tablet   Give _____ tab

4. Ordered: Clonidine 0.6 mg po bid
   On hand: Clonidine 0.3 mg tablet   Give _____ tab

5. Ordered: Ferrous Gluconate 600 mg po bid
   On hand: Ferrous Gluconate 300 mg/5 ml   Give _____ ml

6. Ordered: Zyloprim 100 mg po tid
   On hand: Zyloprim 25 mg tablet   Give _____ tab

7. Ordered: Diphenhydramine 50 mg po q6h
   On hand: Diphenhydramine 12.5 mg/5 ml   Give _____ ml

8. Ordered: Maalox ℥ ss po q 4 hr
   On hand: Maalox liquid   Give _____ ml

9. Ordered: Antivert 25 mg po tid
   On hand: Antivert 10 mg tablet   Give _____ tab

10. Ordered: Elix Phenobarbital 15 mg po q8h
    On hand: Elix Phenobarbital 20 mg/5 ml   Give _____ ml

11. Ordered: Inderal 80 mg po Bid
    On hand: Inderal 20 mg tablet   Give _____ tab

12. Ordered: Lanoxin 0.25 mg po qd
    On hand: Lanoxin 0.125 mg tablet   Give _____ tab

13. Ordered: Guaifenesin 400 mg po q4h
    On hand: Guaifenesin 200 mg/5 ml   Give ____ ml

14. Ordered: Lorazepam 2 mg po bid
    On hand: Lorazepam 0.5 mg tablet   Give ____ tab

15. Ordered: Meclizine 50 mg po tid
    On hand: Meclizine 25 mg tablet   Give ____ tab

16. Ordered: Nilstat 300,000 U po tid
    On hand: Nilstat 100,000 U/ml   Give ____ ml

17. Ordered: Mineral Oil ℥ $\overline{\overline{ii}}$ po after X-ray
    On hand: Mineral Oil 180 ml bottle   Give ____ ml

18. Ordered: Thyroid $\frac{1}{300}$ gr po qd
    On hand: Thyroid 0.2 mg tablet   Give ____ tab

19. Ordered: Niacin 1 g po tid
    On hand: Niacin 250 mg tablet   Give ____ tab

20. Ordered: Pemoline 37.5 mg po daily
    On hand: Pemoline 18.75 mg tablet   Give ____ tab

21. Ordered: Inderal $\frac{2}{3}$ gr po bid
    On hand: Inderal 20 mg capsule   Give ____ cap

22. Ordered: Potassium Chloride 15 mEq po tid
    On Hand: Potassium Chloride 20 mEq/10 ml   Give ____ ml

23. Ordered: Phenergan 12.5 mg po tid
    On hand: Phenergan 25 mg tablet   Give ____ tab

24. Ordered: Ascorbic Acid 500 mg po bid
On hand: Ascorbic Acid 250 mg tablet   Give ____ tab

25. Ordered: Cimetidine 600 mg po q6h
On hand: Cimetidine 200 mg tablet   Give ____ tab

26. Ordered: Colchicine 1.2 mg po
On hand: Colchicine 0.6 mg tablet   Give ____ tab

27. Ordered: Nitroglycerine $\frac{1}{200}$ gr po PRN
On hand: Nitroglycerine 0.6 mg tablet   Give ____ tab

28. Ordered: Elavil 75 mg po H.S.
On hand: Elavil 25 mg tablet   Give ____ tab

29. Ordered: Polycillin 500,000 U po qid
On hand: Polycillin 4,000,000 U/10 ml   Give ____ ml

30. Ordered: Aspirin 0.6 g po q4h
On hand: Aspirin 300 mg tablet   Give ____ tab

31. Ordered: Clindamycin 300 mg po q6h
On hand: Clindamycin 75 mg/5 ml   Give ____ ml

32. Ordered: Mylanta 3 $\overline{ss}$ po q4h
On hand: Mylanta liquid   Give ____ ml

33. Ordered: Elix Phenobarbital gr $\overline{ss}$ po H.S.
On hand: Elix Phenobarbital 100 mg/10 ml   Give ____ ml

34. Ordered: Furosemide 60 mg po daily
On hand: Furosemide 40 mg/ 5 ml   Give ____ ml

35. Ordered: Clinoril 125 mg po bid
On hand: Clinoril 0.5 g tablet   Give ____ tab

36. Ordered: Elix Lanoxin 0.025 mg po qd
On hand: Elix Lanoxin 0.05 mg/5 ml   Give ____ ml

37. Ordered: Diclofenac 150 mg po bid
On hand: Diclofenac 75 mg tablet   Give ____ tab

38. Ordered: Fluoxetine 60 mg po bid
On hand: Fluoxetine 20 mg/5 ml   Give ____ ml

39. Ordered: ASA supp gr x q4h PRN
On hand: ASA supp 300 mg   Give ____ supp

40. Ordered: Rifampin 600 mg po daily
On hand: Rifampin 150 mg capsule   Give ____ cap

41. Give Cefaclor 374 mg from a bottle labeled
Cefaclor 187 mg/5 ml.   Give ____ ml

42. To administer Morphine Sulfate 10 mg from tablets labeled M.S. $\frac{1}{6}$ gr, you would give how many tablets? ____

43. The order reads Elix Phenobarbital 20 mg. Available is a bottle labeled Elix Phenobarbital $\frac{1}{4}$ gr per 5 ml. Correct dose = ____ ml?

44. Ordered is Potassium Chloride 45 mEq po. The label reads KCl 15 mEq/5 ml. You would give ____ ml? ____ ℥?

45. In giving Maalox 30 ml, you would be giving how many ____ ℥?

46. The written order is Valium 2.5 mg. The tablets available are labeled 5 mg. How many tablets would be given? ____ tab

47. Give Inderal 0.24 mg po from a solution labeled Inderal 2 mg per 10 ml. ____ ml

48. The order reads Benadryl 50 mg po. The solution is labeled Benadryl 12.5 mg/5 ml. Amount to give: ____ ml? ____ ℥?

49. The order reads Cortisone 75 mg po. How many tablets would be given from tablets labeled Cortisone 25 mg? ____ tab

50. Give Brethine 10 mg po from tablets labeled Brethine 2.5 mg. ____ tab

51. Give Phenobarbital 60 mg po from tablets labeled Phenobarbital 0.03 g. ____ tab

52. From a bottle labeled Lasix 20 mg per 5 ml, how much would be given to administer Lasix 15 mg? ____ ml

53. The order reads Motrin 0.6 g po. Available are Motrin 600 mg tablets. How many tablets would be given? ____ tab

54. Your unit has Chloral Hydrate 500 mg/5 ml available. The order reads Chloral Hydrate 0.25 g. How many ml will be given? ____ ml

55. The order reads Phenergan 12.5 mg po. The tablets available are labeled Phenergan 25 mg. How many tablets will be given? ____ tab

56. Give Estradiol 0.5 mg from tablets labeled Estradiol 1 mg.

    Give _____ tab

57. The order reads Haloperidol 5 mg po H.S. The bottle is labeled Haloperidol 2 mg/ml. Amount to give: _____ ml.

58. The order reads Keflex 1500 mg po stat. How many g will be given? _____ g

59. Give Nafcillin 1 g from capsules labeled Nafcillin 500 mg.

    Give _____ cap

60. Give Phenobarbital 50 mg po from tablets labeled Phenobarbital $\frac{3}{4}$ gr. _____ tab

61. The order reads Oxaprozin 1800 mg po. Each tablet is labeled Oxaprozin 600 mg. How many tablets will be given?

    Give _____ tab

62. Give Penicillin V 375 mg po from a bottle labeled Penicillin V 125 mg/5 ml.   Give _____ ml

63. Give Primidone 125 mg po from medication labeled Primidone 250 mg/5 ml.   Give _____ ml

64. The order reads Zidovudine 100 mg po. It is available as Zidovudine 50 mg/5 ml. You advise the parent to give the child how many tsp?   Give _____ tsp

65. You have available Lanoxin 0.05 mg per 5 ml. How much would be given to administer Lanoxin 0.125 mg? _____ ml

66. Give Methodone 2.5 mg po from tablets labeled Methodone 5 mg. _____ tab

67. The order reads Tavist 2.68 mg po. Available are tablets labeled Tavist 1.34 mg. How many tablets would be given?

   Give _____ tab

68. Give Cephalexin 1 g po from capsules labeled Cephalexin 250 mg. Give _____ cap

69. On hand is Prednisone 5 mg tablets. The order is to administer Prednisone 0.04 g. _____ tab

70. Give Zyloprim 0.1 g po from tablets labeled Zyloprim 50 mg. _____ tab

71. Available is Codeine 30 mg tablets. How many tablets will be given to administer one gr of Codeine?   Give _____ tab

72. Give Tagamet 0.3 g po from tablets labeled Tagamet 150 mg. _____ tab

73. To administer Mineral Oil ℥ ii po, how many ml would be given? _____ ml

74. Give Lovastatin 60 mg po from tablets labeled Lovastatin 20 mg.

   Give _____ tab

75. Give Sucralfate 1 g po from medication labeled Sucralfate 500 mg/5 ml.   Give _____ ml

ANSWERS

Oral Medications (pp. 94–101)

1. 2 cap	**20.** 2 tab	**39.** 2 supp	**58.** 1.5 Gm
2. 3 tab	**21.** 2 cap	**40.** 4 cap	**59.** 2 cap
3. 4 tab	**22.** 7.5 ml	**41.** 10 ml	**60.** 1 tab
4. 2 tab	**23.** $\frac{1}{2}$ tab	**42.** 1 tab	**61.** 3 tab
5. 10 ml	**24.** 2 tab	**43.** 6.7 ml	**62.** 15 ml
6. 4 tab	**25.** 3 tab	**44.** 15 ml, $\frac{1}{2}$ ʒ	**63.** 2.5 ml
7. 20 ml	**26.** 2 tab	**45.** 1 ʒ	**64.** 2 tsp
8. 15 ml	**27.** $\frac{1}{2}$ tab	**46.** $\frac{1}{2}$ tab	**65.** 12.5 ml
9. $2\frac{1}{2}$ tab	**28.** 3 tab	**47.** 1.2 ml	**66.** $\frac{1}{2}$ tab
10. 3.75 ml	**29.** 1.25 ml	**48.** 20 ml, $\frac{2}{3}$ ʒ	**67.** 2 tab
11. 4 tab	**30.** 2 tab	**49.** 3 tab	**68.** 4 cap
12. 2 tab	**31.** 4 ml	**50.** 4 tab	**69.** 8 tab
13. 10 ml	**32.** 2.5 ml	**51.** 2 tab	**70.** 2 tab
14. 4 tab	**33.** 3 ml	**52.** 3.75 ml	**71.** 2 tab
15. 2 tab	**34.** 7.5 ml	**53.** 1 tab	**72.** 2 tab
16. 3 ml	**35.** $\frac{1}{4}$ tab	**54.** 2.5 ml	**73.** 60 ml
17. 60 ml	**36.** 2.5 ml	**55.** $\frac{1}{2}$ tab	**74.** 3 tab
18. 1 tab	**37.** 2 tab	**56.** $\frac{1}{2}$ tab	**75.** 10 ml
19. 4 tab	**38.** 15 ml	**57.** 2.5 ml	

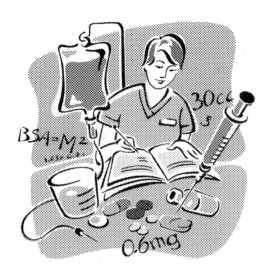

CHAPTER 10

Parenteral Dosages

Parenteral medications are those given by injection. The most common parenteral routes used by nurses are *intradermal, subcutaneous* (or "sub-q"), *intramuscular* (or "IM"), and *intravenous* (or "IV").

Medications given parenterally must be in liquid form to be injected. Some of these medications are prepared as liquids by the manufacturer and are placed into vials or ampules. The label states the amount of medication in a given amount of liquid, as seen below. Other liquid medications are available in either prefilled cartridges for use with reusable plastic or metal syringes or in prefilled syringes, as seen in Figures 10.1 and 10.2. Both cartridges and prefilled syringes are labeled with all necessary information.

Used with permission from Merck and Company, Inc.

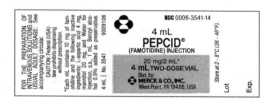

Medications that are unstable as liquids are packaged as powders. The powdered medication must be reconstituted with **sterile diluent** (usually sterile, normal saline or bacteriostatic water). The label on the vial or package insert will tell the amount and type of solution to be mixed with the powder. Carefully follow the manufacturer's guidelines regarding reconstitution. Place the exact amount of diluting solution into the vial. After the powder is dissolved, each ml of liquid will contain a certain concentration of the drug. This information is usually on the drug label as shown on the nafcillin sodium label on p. 104, and is always on the package insert.

FIGURE 10.1 Unassembled, pre-filled cartridges, used with permission from Wyeth-Ayerst Laboratories, St. Davids, PA

FIGURE 10.2 Assembled, pre-filled cartridges, used with permission from Wyeth-Ayerst Laboratories, St. Davids, PA

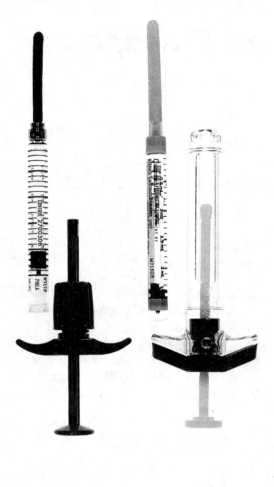

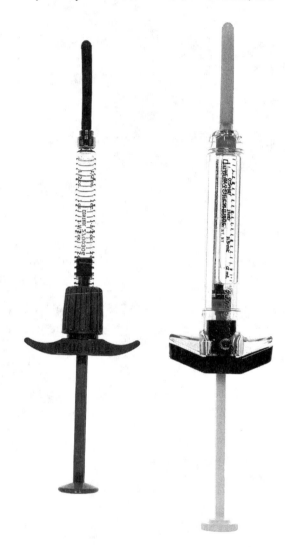

Used with permission from Bristol-Myers Squibb Company

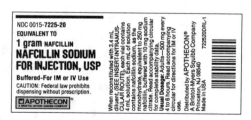

NDC 0015-7225-20
EQUIVALENT TO
1 gram NAFCILLIN
NAFCILLIN SODIUM FOR INJECTION, USP
Buffered-For IM or IV Use
CAUTION: Federal law prohibits dispensing without prescription.
APOTHECON
A BRISTOL-MYERS SQUIBB COMPANY

When reconstituted with 3.4 mL diluent, (SEE INSERT-INTRAMUS-CULAR ROUTE), each vial contains 4 mL solution. Each mL of solution contains nafcillin sodium, as the monohydrate, equivalent to 250 mg nafcillin, buffered with 10 mg sodium citrate. Read accompanying circular for complete stability data.
Usual Dosage: Adults—500 mg every 4 to 6 hours. Read accompanying circular for directions for IM or IV use.
Distributed by APOTHECON®
A Bristol-Myers Squibb Company
Princeton, NJ 08540
Made in USA   7225200RL-1

Parenteral medications may be dispensed in micrograms (mcg), milligrams (mg), grams (g), milliequivalents (mEq), and in units (U). Examples of different preparations of parenteral medications are shown on p. 105.

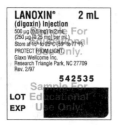

Reproduced with
permission of Glaxo
Wellcome Inc.

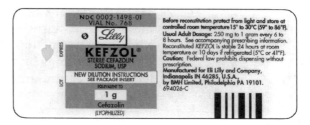

Used with permission from Eli Lilly and
Company, Inc.

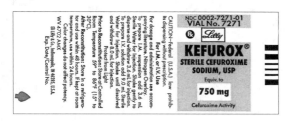

Used with permission from Eli Lilly and
Company, Inc.

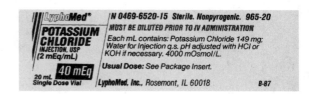

Courtesy LyphoMed, Inc.

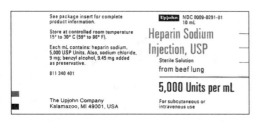

Used with permission from Pharmacia &
Upjohn, Inc.

Syringes are used to administer parenteral medications. Commonly used are the 3 cc (ml) syringe, the 1 cc (ml) or tuberculin syringe, and the insulin syringe.

The markings on the 3 cc (ml) syringe are measured in cc's, (ml) in tenths of a cc, and (ml) in minims.

Three-cc syringe

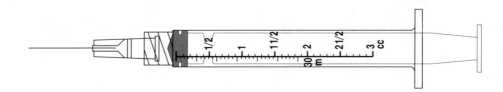

The markings on the tuberculin or 1 cc (ml) syringe are measured in hundredths and tenths of a cc and in minims.

Tuberculin (1 cc)
syringe

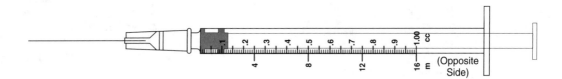

There are two types of insulin syringes. One is a 1 cc (ml) syringe marked off in 100 units. The other is a $\frac{1}{2}$ cc (ml) syringe, which is marked off in 50 units.

Insulin (1 cc) (ml) syringe

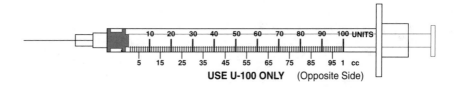

Insulin ($\frac{1}{2}$ cc) (ml) syringe

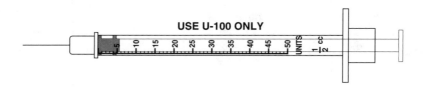

After calculating the amount of medication to be administered, the medication is drawn into the proper syringe and measured as illustrated.

Syringe filled with 2 cc (ml) of medication

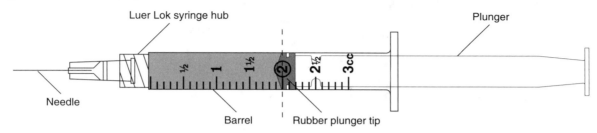

Solving Parenteral Dosages

Parenteral dosage problems can be solved by the ratio and proportion method or by using the formula $\frac{D}{H} \times$ Amount. Remember that when using the formula, D and H must be the same system. We will solve the following problem using both methods.

EXAMPLE: Give Ampicillin 500 mg from a vial labeled Ampicillin 250 mg per 5 cc.

Using the *ratio* and *proportion* method, proceed as follows:

250 mg:5 cc::500 mg: X cc   or $\frac{250 \text{ mg}}{5 \text{ cc}} :: \frac{500 \text{ mg}}{X \text{ cc}}$

$$250\ X \text{ cc} = 2500 \qquad\qquad 250\ X = 2500$$

$$\frac{\overset{1}{\cancel{250}}X \text{ cc}}{\underset{1}{\cancel{250}}} = \frac{\overset{10}{\cancel{2500}}}{\underset{1}{\cancel{250}}} \qquad\qquad X = 10 \text{ cc}$$

$$X = \textbf{10 cc}$$

Using the formula $\frac{D}{H} \times$ *Amount of liquid*, set up the problem as:

$$\frac{\overset{2}{\cancel{500}} \text{ mg}}{\underset{1}{\cancel{250}} \text{ mg}} \times 5 \text{ cc} = \textbf{10 cc}$$

EXAMPLE: The order is for Heparin 7,500 U. Use the label below to solve the problem:

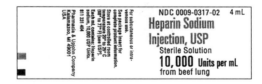

Use the formula $\frac{D}{H} \times$ amount. The amount ordered is the desired dose.

$$\frac{7,500 \text{ U}}{10,000} \times 1 \text{ ml} = 0.75 \text{ ml}$$

PRACTICE PROBLEMS—GIVING PARENTERAL MEDICATIONS FROM RECONSTITUTED POWDERS

The first group of practice problems involve giving parenteral medications from reconstituted powders.

1. Chlorothiazide 750 mg IV is ordered. The drug label states that after reconstitution with 18 ml sterile water, there are 500 mg/10 ml. How many ml should be given? ____ ml

2. Amobarbital 75 mg is ordered IM. When the 250 mg vial is reconstituted, each ml = 100 mg. How much should be administered? ____ ml

3. Give Luecovorin Calcium 1 mg IM. The 50 mg vial label states that when the powder is diluted with 25 ml of sterile water, each ml = 2 mg. How many minims should be administered? ____ m_x

4. Give Kefzol 500 mg IM q6h. Calculate the dosage using the reconstitution instructions on the label. Give ____ ml.

Used with permission from
Eli Lilly and Company, Inc.

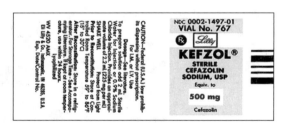

5. Give Methicillin 1 g IM q6h. When the 4 g vial is diluted with 5.7 ml of diluent, each 500 mg = 1 ml. How much should be given to the patient? ____ ml

6. Give Nafcillin 500 mg IM q 6 h. When 3.4 ml of diluent is added to the 1 g vial, 250 mg = 1 ml. What dosage should be given? ____ ml

7. An order reads Oxacillin Sodium IM 500 mg q6h. When 2.8 ml of diluent are added to the 500 mg vial, every 250 mg = 1.5 ml. How much should be administered? _____ ml

8. A drug order is for Cefoperazone 0.5 g IM. When the 2 g vial is diluted with 3.8 ml of sterile diluent, each ml = 250 mg. Give _____ ml.

In the following practice problems, a syringe occasionally will accompany the problem. After calculating the medication dosage, the learner should shade in the amount to be given to the patient.

9. Give Adenosine 8 mg IV push from a vial labeled 6 mg/2 ml. _____ ml

10. Colchicine IV 0.5 mg is ordered. It is available in a vial labeled 500 mcg/ml. Give _____ ml

11. A drug order is for Cortisone Acetate 300 mg IM from a vial labeled 150 mg/ml. Give _____ ml

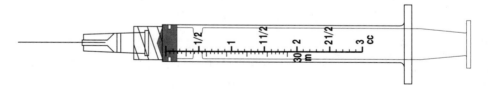

12. Give Dilaudid 0.5 mg IM from a vial labeled 2 mg/ml. Give _____ ml

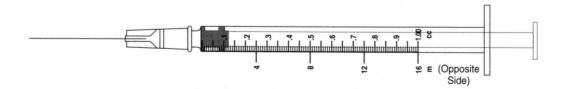

13. Give Amitriptyline 25 mg IM qid from a vial labeled 10 mg/ml. ____ ml

14. A drug order is for Diazepam 2 mg IM from a vial labeled 5 mg/ml. Give ____ ml

15. Give Dimercarprol 125 mg IM. The drug comes in a vial labeled 100 mg/ml. Give ____ ml

16. Give Fentanyl 0.75 mg IV from an ampule labeled 2.5 mg/ml. Give ____ ml

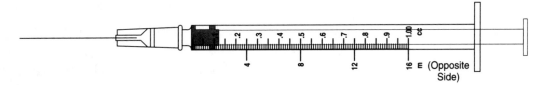

17. The written order is Digoxin 0.5 mg IV. The ampule is labeled 0.25 mg/ml. Give ____ ml

18. Diphenhydramine 12.5 mg IV is ordered. On hand is an ampule labeled 50 mg/ml. How many minims should be given? ____ m_x

19. Give Ephedrine Sulfate 12.5 mg SC from a vial labeled 25 mg/ml. Give ____ ml

20. A drug order is for Epinephrine 0.2 mg sub-q. The drug is available as 1 mg/ml. Give ____ ml

21. Add Potassium Chloride 10 mEq to a bag of IV fluids. The drug is available in a multi-dose vial as labeled on the next page. Withdraw ____ ml.

Courtesy LyphoMed, Inc.

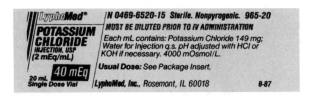

22. Add Bretylium 500 mg to an IV. The drug is available as 50 mg/ml. Give _____ ml

23. A drug order is for Brompheniramine Maleate 10 mg sub-q bid. How many minims should be administered from a vial labeled 100 mg/ml? _____ m$_x$

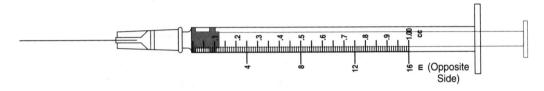

24. Calcitonin 100 U IM is ordered. The vial is labeled 400 U/2 ml. Give _____ ml

25. Give Atropine 0.6 mg IV. The vial is labeled 0.8 mg/ml. Give _____ ml

26. The order is Cefazolin Sodium 250 mg IM q8h. The vial is labeled 500 mg/5 cc. Give _____ cc

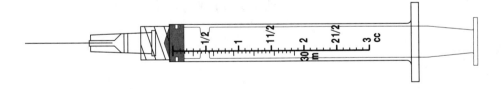

27. Give Aurothioglucose 30 mg IM from a vial labeled 50 mg per ml. _____ ml

28. Bethanechol 2.5 mg SC is ordered tid. The vial is labeled 5 mg/ml. Give _____ ml

29. Give Chlordiazepoxide 50 mg IV tid. The vial is labeled 100 mg/2 ml. _____ ml

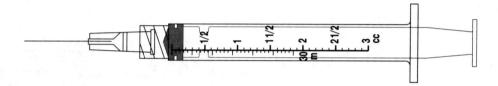

30. Give Amikacin 250 mg IM. The vial is labeled 0.25 g per ml. _____ ml

31. Give Butorphanol 0.5 mg IV. The drug is available as 2 mg/ml. _____ ml

32. Carboprost 200 mcg is ordered. The drug is available as 250 mcg/ml. Give _____ ml

33. Give Clindamycin 300 mg IM. The vial is labeled 150 mg per ml. Give _____ ml

34. Glucagon 0.5 mg IM is ordered. On hand is a 10-mg vial. The vial reads 1 mg/ml. _____ ml

35. Give Pepcid 5 mg IV. Use the label to calculate the dosage. Give _____ ml

Used with permission from
Merck and Company, Inc.

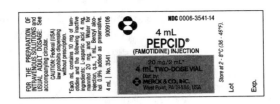

36. The order reads Methylprednisolone Sodium 25 mg IV. The vial is labeled 0.05 g/5 ml. _____ ml

37. Furosemide 20 mg IV is ordered. It is available as 10 mg/ml. Give _____ ml

38. Give Nafcillin 500 mg IM q6h. When 3.4 ml of diluent is added to the 1 g vial, 250 mg = 1 ml. What dosage is given? _____ ml

39. Give Oxymorphone 1 mg IM. It is available as 1.5 mg/ml. Administer _____ ml

40. Give Penicillin G Potassium 1,000,000 U IM q6h. The vial label reads 500,000 U per 1 cc. _____ ml

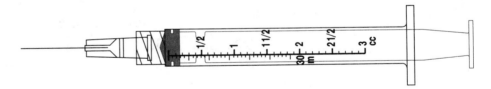

41. Give Protamine Sulfate 25 mg IV. The vial is labeled 10 mg/ml. _____ ml

42. Give Phenylephrine 2.5 mg SC. The drug is available as 10 mg/ml. Give _____ ml

The next group of problems are anesthesia (pre-op) orders. In each case, you must calculate the amount of each medication and decide if you need one or two 3-cc syringes to draw the total medication. *The drugs in these practice problems are compatible and can be mixed together.*

43. Give 0.1 mg Robinul
    25 mg Benadryl   ⟩IM on call to OR
    75 mg Meperidine
    On hand, there is Robinul 0.2 mg/ml
                      Benadryl 50 mg/ml
                      Meperidine 100 mg/2 ml

    Robinul ____ ml
    Benadryl ____ ml
    Meperidine ____ ml
    Syringe(s) ____

44. Give Phenergan 25 mg and Morphine 8 mg IM as a pre-op. Phenergan is available as 50 mg/ml and Morphine is available as $\frac{1}{6}$ gr per 2 ml.

    Phenergan ____ ml
    Morphine ____ ml
    Syringe(s) ____

45. A pre-op order reads Dilaudid 1 mg, Benadryl 25 mg, Robinul 0.2 mg. On hand is: Dilaudid 2 mg/ml
                      Benadryl 50 mg/ml
                      Robinul 0.2 mg/ml

    Dilaudid ____ ml   Benadryl ____ ml   Robinul ____ ml
    Syringe(s) ____

46. Give Demerol 50 mg, Versed 2 mg, and Robinul 0.1 mg as a pre-op. Available is Demerol 100 mg/2 ml, Versed 1 mg/ml and Robinul 0.2 mg/ml.

    ____ ml Demerol   ____ ml Robinul
    ____ ml Versed   ____ Syringe(s)

47. Give a child Meperidine 15 mg and Atropine 0.1 mg IM prior to surgery. The drugs come as Meperidine 50 mg/ml and Atropine 0.4 mg/ml.

    Meperidine ____ ml
    Atropine ____ ml
    Syringe(s) ____

48. A pre-op order is for Reglan 10 mg and Versed 1 mg. The drugs are available as:

Reglan 5 mg/ml   Give ____ ml
Versed 2 mg/2 ml   Give ____ ml
Syringe(s) ____

49. Give Benadryl 25 mg
      Atropine 0.2 mg   ⟩ IM on call to OR
      Morphine 4 mg

On hand is Benadryl 50 mg/ml, Atropine 0.4 mg/ml, and Morphine 8 mg/ml.

____ ml Benadryl   ____ ml Atropine   ____ ml Morphine
____ Syringe(s)

50. Give Dilaudid 1.5 mg and Versed 0.75 mg IM on call. The drugs are on hand as:

Dilaudid 2 mg/ml   Give ____ ml
Versed 2 mg/2 ml   Give ____ ml
                       Syringe(s) ____

51. Give the following pre-op: Meperdine 100 mg
                              Atropine 0.6 mg
                              Benadryl 12.5 mg
Available is: Meperidine 50 mg/ml ____ ml
                     Atropine 0.6 mg/ml ____ ml
                     Benadryl 50 mg/ml ____ ml
                     Syringe(s) ____

52. A pre-op order for a pregnant patient is for Meperidine 50 mg and Robinul 0.2 mg. Available is Meperidine 50 mg/ml and Robinul 0.4 mg/2 mg.

____ ml Meperidine   ____ ml Robinul
____ Syringe(s)

The next group of practice problems deal with drugs typically measured in units per ml. Units are abbreviated as U.

53. Heparin 5000 U is ordered. The vial is labeled 10,000 U per ml.
Give ____ m$_x$

Used with permission from
Merck and Company, Inc.

54. Give Decadron 3 mg from a vial as labeled below. _____ ml

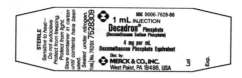

55. Give Heparin 2500 U from a 10,000 U/ml vial. _____ ml

56. Give Potassium Penicillin G 1,000,000 U from a vial labeled 10,000,000 U/10 ml. _____ ml

57. Give Heparin 7500 U from a vial labeled 5000 U/ml. _____ ml

58. Give Penicillin G 100,000 U from a vial of 1,000,000 U per 5 ml. _____ ml

59. Administer Heparin 20,000 U sub-q q6h. The vial is labeled 10,000 U/ml. Give _____ ml

60. Give Procaine Penicillin 400,000 U from a vial labeled 150,000 U per cc. _____ cc

61. Give Heparin 15,000 U IV from a vial labeled Heparin 1,000 U/ml. _____ ml

62. Give Penicillin G Benzathine 1,200,000 U from a vial of 600,000 U/ml. _____ ml

The next group of practice problems deals with drugs commonly dispensed as *mg/ml or mcg/ml.*

63. Give Betamethasone Sodium 12 mg IV qd. The drug is available as 6 mg/ml. Give _____ ml

64. The order is for Chloroquine 160 mg IM qd. It is available as 50 mg/ml. ____ ml

65. Give Aminophylline 125 mg IV q6h from a vial labeled 0.25 g/10 ml. ____ ml

66. Administer Lanoxin 125 mcg IM daily. Calculate dose using the label below. ____ ml

Reproduced with permission of Glaxo Wellcome Inc.

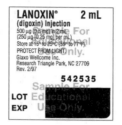

67. A drug order is for Chlorpheniramine 15 mg IM. The drug is available as 10 mg/ml. ____ ml

68. Give Chlorpromazine 50 mg IM q12h from a vial labeled 25 mg/ml. ____ ml

69. Give Cimetidine HCL 150 mg q4h IM. The drug is available as 300 mg/2 ml. ____ ml

70. Give Ethylnorepinephrine 1 mg sub-q from a vial labeled 2 mg/ml. ____ m_x

71. A drug order is for Fluorouracil 400 mg IV. The drug is available as 50 mg/ml. ____ ml

72. Give Lasix 40 mg IV from a vial labeled 10 mg/ml. ____ ml

73. The order is for Gentamicin 50 mg IM tid. The drug is available as 40 mg/ml. _____ ml

74. A drug order is for Gold Sodium Thiomalate 5 mg IM. The drug comes in a vial labeled 25 mg/ml. _____ ml

75. Give Haloperidol 3 mg from a vial labeled 5 mg/ml. _____ ml

76. The order is for Imipramine HC1 25 mg IM tid. The drug is available as 12.5 mg per ml. _____ ml

77. Give Isoniazid 150 mg IM from a vial labeled 100 mg/ml. _____ ml

78. The order is for Kanamycin 250 mg q6h IM. The drug is available as 500 mg/2 ml. _____ ml

79. Give Leuprolide 7.5 mg IM from a vial labeled 5 mg/ml. _____ ml

80. The order is for Demerol 75 mg q4h IM prn. The drug is available as 100 mg/2 ml. _____ ml

81. A drug order is for Mesoridiazine Besylate 25 mg IM. The drug is available as 0.25 g/ml. _____ ml

82. Give Methadone 2.5 mg sub-q from a vial labeled 10 mg per ml. _____ ml

83. A drug order is for Methocarbamol 1 g IV q 8 h. The drug is available as 100 mg/ml. _____ ml

84. Give Methyldopate 750 mg IV from a vial labeled 250 mg per 5 ml. _____ ml

85. The order is for Methylprednisolone Acetate 25 mg IM. The drug is available in a vial containing 40 mg per ml. Give _____ m_x

86. The order reads Miconazole 200 mg IV. It is available in a vial containing 10 mg per ml. Give _____ ml

87. Give Morphine Sulfate $\frac{1}{12}$ gr from an ampule containing 10 mg per ml. Give _____ m_x

88. Give Naloxone 0.01 mg IV from a vial labeled 20 mcg per ml. _____ ml

89. The written order is Neomycin 400 mg IM. The drug is available as 500 mg per 2.5 ml. _____ ml

90. Physostigmine 500 mcg IV is ordered. The drug is available as 1 mg per ml. _____ ml

91. Give Oxytetracycline 100 mg IM q8h. The drug is in a vial labeled 125 mg per ml. _____ ml

92. Give Phenylephrine 2.5 mg SC. The drug is available as 10 mg/ml. _____ ml

The following problems are on insulin dosage. Insulin is prepared as 100 U per ml. Several pharmaceutical companies manufacture different types of insulin, but all are 100 U per ml and are labeled U-100. An insulin syringe is used to draw the correct dosage. If 50 U or less are needed, the $\frac{1}{2}$ cc 50-unit syringe may be used. The 1 cc 100-unit syringe may be used for any dosage up to 100 units. In the problems beginning below, the student is to shade in the correct amount of insulin to be drawn into the syringe.

Used with permission from Eli Lilly and Company, Inc.

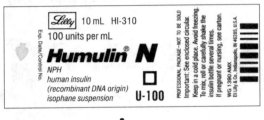

A

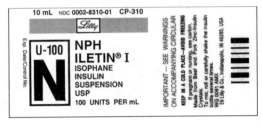

B

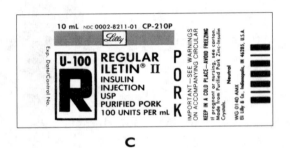

C

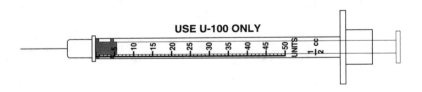

D

93. Humulin R 16 U sub-q every morning.

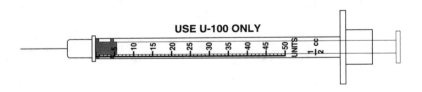

94. Novolin N 48 U sub-q before breakfast.

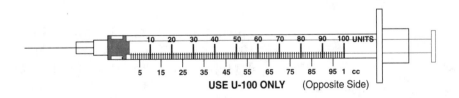

95. NPH Iletin II 38 U sub-q at 4 P.M.

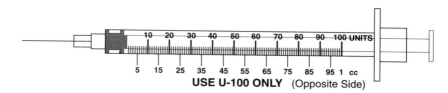

96. Novolin R 5 U IV now.

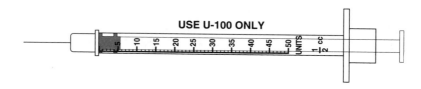

97. Humulin R 10 U and Humulin N 25 U sub-q at 7:30 A.M. (Mix in the same syringe.)

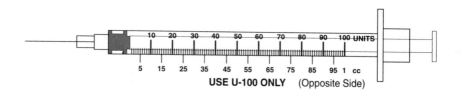

ANSWERS

Giving Parenteral Medications from Reconstituted Powders (pp. 108–121)

1. 15 ml	**6.** 2 ml
2. 0.75 ml	**7.** 3 ml
3. 8 m$_x$	**8.** 2 ml
4. 2.2 ml	**9.** 2.7 ml
5. 2 ml	**10.** 1 ml

11. 2 ml

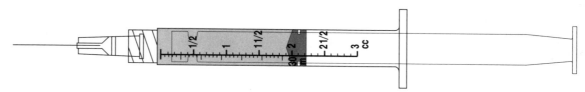

12. 0.25 ml

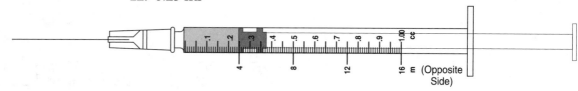

13. 2.5 ml   **15.** 1.25 ml
14. 0.4 ml

16. 0.3 ml

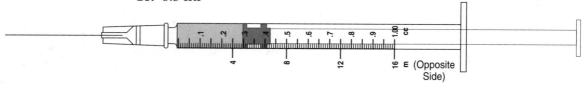

17. 2 ml   **20.** 0.2 ml
18. 4 m$_x$ **21.** 7.5 ml
19. 0.5 ml   **22.** 10 ml

23. 2 m$_x$

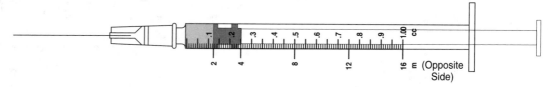

24. 0.5 ml   **25.** 0.75 ml

26. 2.5 cc

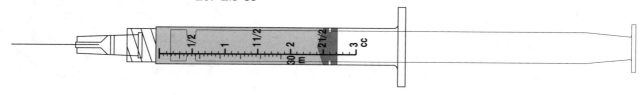

27. 0.6 ml   **28.** 0.5 ml

29. 1 ml

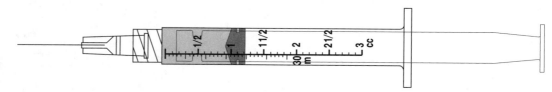

30. 1 ml

31. 0.25 ml

32. 0.8 ml

33. 2 ml

34. 0.5 ml

35. 0.5 ml

36. 2.5 ml

37. 2 ml

38. 2 ml

39. 0.7 ml or 0.67 ml

40. 2 ml

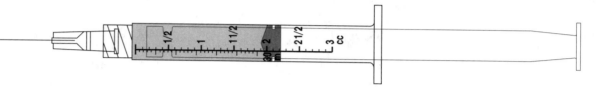

41. 2.5 ml

42. 0.25 ml

43. Robinul 0.5 ml
Benadryl 0.5 ml
Meperidine 1.5 ml
Syringes 1

44. Phenergan 0.5 ml
Morphine 1.6 ml
Syringes 1

45. Dilaudid 0.5 ml
Benadryl 0.5 ml
Robinul 1 ml
Syringes 1

46. Demerol 1 ml
Versed 2 ml
Robinul 0.5 ml
Syringes 2

47. Meperidine 0.3 ml
Atropine 0.25 ml
Syringes 1

48. Reglan 2 ml
Versed 1 ml
Syringes 1

49. Benadryl 0.5 ml
Atropine 0.5 ml
Morphine 0.5 ml
Syringes 1

50. Dilaudid 0.75 ml
Versed 0.75 ml
Syringes 1

51. Meperidine 2 ml
Atropine 1 ml
Benadryl 0.25 ml
Syringes 2

52. Meperidine 1 ml
Robinul 1 ml
Syringes 1

53. 8 m_x

54. 0.75 ml

55. 0.25 ml

56. 1 ml

57. 1.5 ml

58. 0.5 ml

59. 2 ml

60. 2.7 ml

61. 15 ml

62. 2 ml

63. 2 ml

64. 3.2 ml

65. 5 ml

66. 0.5 ml

67. 1.5 ml

68. 2 ml

69. 1 ml

70. 8 m$_x$

71. 8 ml

72. 4 ml

73. 1.25 ml

74. 0.2 ml

75. 0.6 ml

76. 2 ml

77. 1.5 ml

78. 1 ml

79. 1.5 ml

80. 1.5 ml

81. 0.1 ml

82. 0.25 ml

83. 10 ml

84. 15 ml

85. 10 m$_x$

86. 20 ml

87. 8 m$_x$

88. 0.5 ml

89. 2 ml

90. 0.5 ml

91. 0.8 ml

92. 0.25 ml

93.

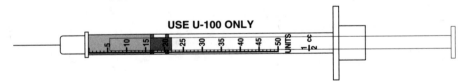

94.

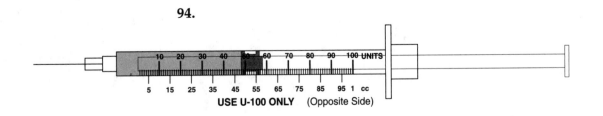

95.

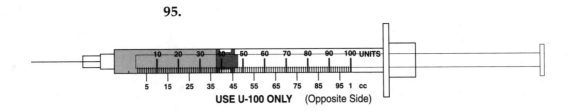

96.

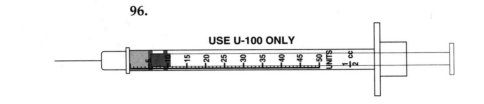

97.

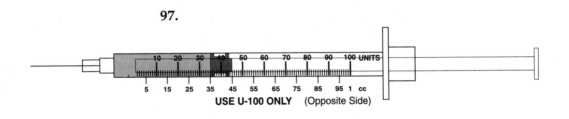

CHAPTER 11

IV Calculation

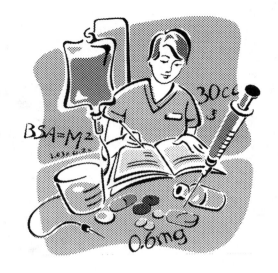

The prescriber should order the type and amount of IV fluid, but it is generally a nurse's responsibility to calculate the rate of infusion. The order should always include the amount of fluid and the number of hours it should be administered. IV administration sets are predetermined by the manufacturer to deliver a certain number of drops per ml (drop factor). Nursing personnel should refer to the administration set label if they are unfamiliar with the drop factor of the set being used. Standard IV administration sets vary in calibration, from 10 drops/ml to 20 drops/ml, depending on the manufacturer.

In this chapter, you will be working with the following administration sets:

$$\text{Microdrip} = 60 \text{ drops (gtt) per ml}$$
$$\text{Standard IV set} = 15 \text{ drops (gtt) per ml}$$
$$\text{Blood administration set} = 10 \text{ drops (gtt) per ml}$$

Calculation of IV Fluids

REMEMBER

The formula for calculating IV infusion rates is:

$$\frac{\text{Amount of fluid (in ml)}}{\text{Time in min}} \times \frac{\text{Administration}}{\text{set drop factor}} = \frac{\text{Drops}}{\text{per min}}$$

EXAMPLE: To administer 500 ml of IV fluid over 8 hr using a microdrip administration set, how many gtt/min would you administer?

$$\frac{500 \text{ ml (amount in ml)}}{480 \text{ (time in min)}} \times 60 \text{ (administration set drop factor)}$$

$$= 104 \times 60 = \textbf{62 gtt/min}$$

EXAMPLE: Give 450 ml of whole blood over 3 hr, using a blood administration set. How many gtts/min will be given?

$$\frac{450 \text{ (amount in ml)}}{180 \text{ (time in minutes)}} = 2.5 \times 10 \text{ (adm. set gtt factor)}$$

$$= \textbf{25 gtts/min}$$

PRACTICE PROBLEMS—CALCULATION OF IV FLUIDS

Note: Round your answer off to the nearest whole number:

	Amount	*Time*	*IV Set Drop Factor*	*Gtt/Min*
1.	225 ml	3 hr	15	_____
2.	1200 ml	12 hr	60	_____
3.	125 ml	1 hr	15	_____
4.	250 ml	2 hr	60	_____
5.	2400 ml	8 hr	15	_____
6.	450 ml	6 hr	10	_____
7.	500 ml	4 hr	60	_____
8.	100 ml	2 hr	15	_____
9.	1500 ml	3 hr	10	_____
10.	2400 ml	12 hr	15	_____
11.	150 ml	1 hr	15	_____

	Amount	Time	IV Set Drop Factor	Gtt/Min
12.	58 ml	1 hr	60	____
13.	400 ml	4 hr	60	____
14.	1000 ml	8 hr	15	____
15.	1200 ml	12 hr	15	____
16.	200 ml	1 hr	10	____
17.	750 ml	3 hr	10	____
18.	24 ml	1 hr	60	____
19.	150 ml	1 hr	10	____
20.	1000 ml	12 hr	60	____
21.	500 ml	24 hr	60	____
22.	1500 ml	12 hr	10	____
23.	20 ml	1 hr	60	____
24.	650 ml	2 hr	15	____
25.	1600 ml	8 hr	15	____

	Amount	Time	IV Set Drop Factor	Gtt/Min
26.	4000 ml	24 hr	15	____
27.	700 ml	4 hr	60	____
28.	1200 ml	24 hr	60	____
29.	800 ml	8 hr	60	____
30.	75 ml	1 hr	60	____
31.	550 ml	2 hr	15	____
32.	375 ml	3 hr	10	____
33.	16 ml	1 hr	60	____
34.	320 ml	4 hr	15	____
35.	1400 ml	8 hr	10	____
36.	1000 ml	4 hr	10	____
37.	900 ml	12 hr	15	____
38.	675 ml	3 hr	15	____
39.	600 ml	8 hr	60	____

	Amount	Time	IV Set Drop Factor	Gtt/Min
40.	3000 ml	24 hr	60	____

41. Infuse D_5W 1000 ml in 8 hr, using a standard IV set. ____ gtt/min

42. Infuse Ringer's Lactate 1500 ml over 12 hr, using a standard IV set. ____ gtt/min

43. Infuse Ionosol MB 500 ml over 8 hr, using a microdrip IV set. ____ gtt/min

44. Infuse $D_5 \frac{1}{2}$ NS 3000 ml continuously qd, using a standard IV set. ____ gtt/min

45. Infuse 1 U whole blood (500 ml) over 4 hr, using a blood administration set. ____ gtt/min

46. Infuse $D_5 \frac{1}{4}$ NS 300 ml over 4 hr, using a microdrip IV set. ____ gtt/min

47. Infuse D_5 Ringer's Lactate 500 ml over 4 hr, using a microdrip IV set. ____ gtt/min

48. An order reads 1000 ml Normosol M over 12 hr. Using a standard IV set, regulate the fluid at ____ gtt/min.

49. An order reads 500 ml $D_5 \frac{1}{4}$ NS to infuse at 30 ml per hr. Using a microdrip IV set, regulate the fluid at ____ gtt/min.

50. Infuse 250 ml packed red cells over 4 hr, using a blood administration IV set. ____ gtt/min

51. An order reads 500 ml D$_5$W to infuse at 50 ml per hr. Using a standard IV set, regulate the fluid at _____ gtt/min.

52. Infuse 1000 ml normal saline $\frac{1}{2}$ % at 75 ml per hr. Using a standard IV set, regulate the rate at _____ gtt/min.

53. A two-month-old infant is ordered to receive 250 ml D$_5$ $\frac{1}{4}$ NS at 5 ml per hr. Using a microdrip set, regulate rate at _____ gtt/min.

54. A patient on hyperalimentation fluid is ordered to receive 500 ml at 83 ml per hour. Using a standard IV set, regulate the rate at _____ gtt/min.

55. An order reads D$_5$ NS 1000 ml to infuse over 24 hr. Using a standard IV set, regulate the rate at _____ gtt/min.

56. Give 50 ml whole blood over 2 hr. Use a blood administration IV set, and regulate the rate at _____ gtt/min.

57. Infuse D$_5$ $\frac{1}{2}$ NS 1000 ml at 175 ml per hour. Use a standard IV set. Regulate the rate at _____ gtt/min.

58. A patient's hyperalimentation fluid is to infuse at 63 ml per hour. Using a microdrip set, regulate the rate at _____ gtt/min.

59. D$_5$ $\frac{1}{4}$ NS is ordered at KVO (keep vein open) rate, not to exceed 20 ml/hour. Using a microdrip IV set, regulate the rate at _____ gtt/min.

60. An order reads TPN 2000 ml to infuse over 24 hr. Using a standard IV set, regulate the rate at _____ gtt/min.

61. Infuse 300 ml plasma over 8 hr using a blood administration IV set. Regulate the rate at _____ gtt/min.

62. Infuse 600 ml Normosol R over 12 hr using a microdrip IV set. Regulate the rate at _____ gtt/min.

63. Infuse 1800 ml D_5 Lactated Ringer's over 24 hr. Use a standard IV set. Regulate the rate at _____ gtt/min.

64. Infuse 150 ml whole blood over 2 hr. Use a blood administration IV set. Regulate the rate at _____ gtt/min.

65. Infuse 400 ml $D_5 \frac{1}{2}$ NS over 4 hr. Using a microdrip IV set, regulate the rate at _____ gtt/min.

66. An order reads 100 ml $D_5 \frac{1}{4}$ NS to infuse at 50 ml/hr for 2 hr. Using a microdrip IV set, regulate the rate at _____ gtt/min.

67. Infuse 1000 ml NS at 200 ml/hr. Using a standard IV set, regulate the rate at _____ gtt/min.

68. An order reads Lactated Ringer's 1000 ml to infuse at 140 ml/hr. Using a standard IV set, regulate the rate at _____ gtt/min.

69. Infuse packed red cells 450 ml over 3 hr. Using a blood administration set, regulate the rate at _____ gtt/min.

70. An order reads Normosol M 1000 ml to infuse at 75 ml/hr. Using a microdrip IV set, regulate the rate at _____ gtt/min.

71. Infuse 3000 ml D$_5\frac{1}{4}$ NS over 12 hr. Using a standard IV set, regulate the rate at ____ gtt/min.

72. Infuse 300 ml whole blood over 4 hr. Using a blood administration set, regulate the rate at ____ gtt/min.

73. An order reads 1200 ml D$_5$W to infuse over 8 hr. Using standard IV set, regulate the rate at ____ gtt/min.

74. Infuse D$_5\frac{1}{2}$ NS 1000 ml at 42 ml/hr. Using a microdrip IV set, regulate the rate at ____ gtt/min.

75. Infuse 600 ml Normosol M over 8 hr. Using a standard IV set, regulate the rate at ____ gtt/min.

76. An order reads 75 ml packed red cells to infuse over 3 hr. Using a blood administration set, regulate the rate at ____ gtt/min.

77. Infuse 2400 ml of IV fluid qd. Using a standard IV set, regulate the rate at ____ gtt/min.

78. An order reads 150 ml of D$_5$W to infuse over 3 hr. Using a blood administration set, regulate the rate at ____ gtt/min.

Calculation of IV Drugs (Titration)

Some drugs given intravenously are potent and may affect the patient quickly and dramatically. These drugs are given by titrating the dosage; that is, increasing or decreasing the amount of drug given until the desired effect has been achieved (for example, raising or lowering the blood pressure). To ensure that the proper dosage is administered, an IV infusion pump is used. These machines are calibrated to deliver a specific amount in ml/hr.

SOLVE MCG/KG/MIN OR HR

STEPS

1. Convert weight to kg if necessary (2.2 lb = 1 kg).

2. Determine strength of solution (mcg/ml).

3. Multiply the strength of solution (mcg/ml) by the rate of infusion.

4. Divide mcg/hr by kg of body weight.

5. Divide mcg/kg/hr by 60 to convert hours to minutes, if necessary.

EXAMPLE: A patient is receiving a drug which has been titrated for effect at 9 ml/hr. The drug is available as 500 mg/500 ml of fluid. The patient weighs 132 lb. How many mcg/kg/min is the patient receiving?

Step 1:   Convert lb to kg.

$$\frac{2.2 \text{ lb}}{\text{kg}} = \frac{132}{X} \qquad\qquad 2.2\,X = 132$$

$$X = \frac{132}{2.2}$$

$$X = 60 \text{ kg}$$

Step 2:   Determine the strength of solution (mcg or mg/ml).

$$\frac{500 \text{ mg}}{500 \text{ ml}} = \frac{1 \text{ mg}}{1 \text{ ml}} = \frac{1000 \text{ mcg}}{1 \text{ ml}}$$

Step 3:   Multiply strength of solution by the rate of infusion.

$$1000 \text{ mcg/ml} \times 9 \text{ ml/hr} = 9000 \text{ mcg/hr}$$

Step 4:   Divide mcg/ml by kg of body weight.

$$\frac{9000 \text{ mcg/hr}}{60 \text{ kg}} = 150 \text{ mcg/kg/hr}$$

Step 5:   Divide mcg/kg/hr by 60 to change hours to minutes.

$$\frac{150 \text{ mcg/kg/hr}}{60} = 2.5 \text{ mcg/kg/min}$$

Answer: 2.5 mcg/kg/min

EXAMPLE: A patient who weighs 60 kg is receiving a drug that has been titrated for effect at 60 ml/hr. The drug is mixed as 500 mg per 1000 ml of fluid. The physician asks, "How many mcg/kg/min is the patient receiving?"

Step 1:   Weight = 60 kg
Step 2:   Determine strength of solution.

$$\frac{500\ mg}{1000\ ml} = \frac{0.5\ mg}{1\ ml} = \frac{500\ mcg}{1\ ml}$$

Step 3:   Multiply the strength of solution by the rate of infusion.

$$500\ mcg/ml \times 60 = 30{,}000\ mcg/hr$$

Step 4:   Divide mcg/hr by kg of body weight.

$$\frac{30{,}000\ mcg/hr}{60\ kg} = 500\ mcg/kg/hr$$

Step 5:   Divide mcg/kg/hr by 60 to change hours to minutes.

$$\frac{500\ mcg/kg/hr}{60} = 8.33\ mcg/kg/min$$

Answer: 8.33 mcg/kg/min

In another type problem, you will be given an amount of medication per kg of body weight to administer per minute or per hour. You will also be asked to determine the infusion pump rate.

REMEMBER

Infusion pumps deliver in ml/hr.

SOLVE MCG/MIN OR HOUR AND INFUSION RATE

EXAMPLE: Give Dopamine 10 mcg/kg/min from a solution that is

STEPS

1. Convert weight to kg if necessary.
2. Multiply dose ordered by the kg of body weight.
3. Multiply mcg/min by 60 to change minutes to hours.
4. To determine rate of infusion:
   a. Determine strength of solution.
   b. Divide strength of solution into amount of medication to be given/per hour.

$$\frac{Desired\ dose\ (mcg/hr)}{Amount\ on\ hand\ (strength\ of\ solution)} = ml/hr$$

mixed 400 mg in 250 ml of fluid. The patient weighs 140 lb. How many mcg/min will you give? Mcg/hr? What will the infusion rate be?

Step 1: Convert lb to kg.

$$\frac{2.2\ lb}{kg} = \frac{140}{X} \qquad\qquad 2.2\ X = 140$$

$$X = \frac{140}{2.2}$$

$$X = 63.63\ kg$$

Step 2: Multiply dose ordered by kg of body weight.

63.63 kg × 10 − 636.3 mcg/min

Step 3: Multiply mcg/min by 60 to change minutes to hours.

636.3 mcg/min × 60 = 38,178.0 mcg/hr

Step 4: Determine the infusion rate.
  a. Determine strength of solution
  b. Divide strength of solution into amount of medication/hr.

$$\frac{400\ mg}{250\ ml} = \frac{1.6\ mg}{1\ ml} = \frac{1600\ mcg}{1\ ml}$$

$$\frac{D}{H} = \frac{38,178\ mcg/hr}{1600\ mcg/ml} = 23.8 = 24\ ml/hr.$$

Answers: 636.3 mcg/min
38,178 mcg/hr; Rate = 24 ml/hr.

REMEMBER

Infusion pump rates should always be rounded to whole numbers, unless you are using a micro pump.

EXAMPLE: Infuse a drug at 5 mcg/kg/min to a patient weighing 165 lb. The drug is mixed 250 mg in 250 ml of fluid. How many mcg/min will you give? mcg/hr? What will the rate of infusion be?

Step 1: Convert weight to kg.

$$\frac{2.2\ lb}{kg} = \frac{165}{X} \qquad\qquad 2.2\ X = 165$$

$$X = \frac{165}{2.2}$$

$$X = 75\ kg$$

Step 2: Multiply dose by kg of body weight.

75 kg × 5 mcg = 375 mcg/min

Step 3: Multiply mcg/min by 60 to change minutes to hours.

375 mcg/min × 60 = 22,500 mcg/hr

Step 4: Determine the infusion rate.
      a. Determine strength of solution.
      b. Divide strength of solution into amount of medication/hr.

$$\frac{250 \text{ mg}}{250 \text{ ml}} = \frac{1 \text{ mg}}{1 \text{ ml}} = \frac{1000 \text{ mcg}}{1 \text{ ml}}$$

$$\frac{D}{H} = \frac{22500 \text{ mcg/hr}}{1000 \text{ mcg/ml}} = 22.5 = 23 \text{ ml/hr}$$

Answers: 375 mcg/min   22,500 mcg/hr   23 ml/hr.

Consider this somewhat different problem:

Add 2 g of Lidocaine to 500 ml of fluid and infuse at a rate of 2 mg per min. At what rate should the infusion pump be set per hour?

Step 1: Determine strength of solution.

$$\frac{2 \text{ g}}{500 \text{ ml}} = \frac{2000 \text{ mg}}{500 \text{ ml}} = \frac{4 \text{ mg}}{1 \text{ ml}}$$

Step 2: Divide strength of solution into amount of medication ordered.

$$\frac{2 \text{ mg/min}}{4 \text{ mg}} = 0.5 \text{ ml/min}$$

Step 3: Multiply ml/min by 60 to change minutes to hours.

$$0.5 \text{ ml} \times 60 = 30 \text{ ml/hr}$$

Answer: Rate = 30 ml/hr.

PRACTICE PROBLEMS—TITRATION

Solve:

1. A patient who weighs 50 kg is receiving an Aminophylline drip at the rate of 50 ml/hr. The drug is available as 250 mg/500 ml of fluid. How many mcg/kg/min is the patient receiving?

    _____ mcg/kg/min

2. A patient is receiving Inocar that has been titrated for effect at 9 ml/hr. The drug is mixed as 500 mg/500 ml of fluid. If the patient weighs 60 kg, how many mcg/kg/min is he receiving?

    _____ mcg/kg/min

3. Give Nitroprusside 0.5 mcg/kg/min to a patient weighing 80 kg. The drug is mixed 500 mg/500 ml D_5 W. How many mcg/hr will he receive? What will the infusion pump rate be?

    _____ mcg/hr   _____ ml/hr

4a. Aminophylline 5.6 mg/kg is given as a loading dose over 20 minutes. The drug is mixed 250 mg/250 ml D_5 W. If the patient's weight is 110 lb, how many mg/dose will you give?

_____ mg/dose

4b. After the loading dose has been given, Aminophylline 0.8 mg/kg/hr is ordered for this patient. Using the same mixture of medication, how many mg/hr will you give? What is the infusion pump rate?

_____ mg/hr   _____ ml/hr

5. A patient is receiving Brevibloc at the rate of 30 ml/hr. If the drug is mixed as 5 g in 500 ml of fluid and the patient weighs 100 kg, how many mcg/kg/hr is the patient receiving?

_____ mcg/kg/hr

6. Aminophylline 50 mg/hr is ordered. The drug is available as 1 g/500 ml of fluid. At what rate should the infusion pump be programmed per hour?

_____ ml/hr

7. Administer Dopamine at a rate of 10 ml/hr to a patient who weighs 110 lb. The drug is available as 800 mg, added to 1000 ml of fluid. How many mcg/kg/hr will the patient receive?

_____ mcg/kg/hr

8. Give Lidocaine 30 mcg/kg/min to a child weighing 55 lb. The drug is available as 120 mg/100 ml of fluid. How many mcg/min will be given? Mcg/hr? What will be the infusion pump rate?

_____ mcg/min   _____ mcg/hr   _____ ml/hr

9. Heparin 16 U/kg/hr is ordered. It is mixed 5000 U/250 ml of fluid. The patient weighs 145 lb. How many U will be given per minute. What will the infusion pump rate be?

_____ U/min   _____ ml/hr

10. A patient weighing 166 lb is receiving a drug which has been titrated for effect at 30 ml/hr. The drug is mixed as 250 mg/500 ml of fluid. How many mcg/kg/min is the patient receiving?

    _____ mcg/kg/min

11. A patient weighing 170 lb is to receive Norepinephrine 4 mg/1000 ml D_5 W at 42 ml/hr. How many mcg/kg/min will he receive? How many mcg/kg/hr?

    _____ mcg/kg/min   _____ mcg/kg/hr

12. Give Aminophylline 20 mg/hr. If the drug is available as 1 g/500 ml of fluid, at what rate should the infusion run per hour?

    _____ ml/hr

13. A patient is receiving a drug at the rate of 40 ml/hr. The drug is mixed 200 mg/250 ml of fluid. If the patient weighs 80 lb, how many mcg/kg/min is being delivered?

    _____ mcg/kg/min

14. Inocar has been titrated for effect at 12 ml/hr. The drug is mixed 300 mg/250 ml of fluid. The patient weighs 80 kg. How many mcg/kg/min is the patient receiving?

    _____ mcg/kg/min

15. You are to give Lidocaine 0.027 mg/kg/min to a patient weighing 172 lb. The drug is available as 2 g/500 ml of D_5 W. How many mg/min will you give? Mg/hr? What will the infusion rate be?

    _____ mg/min   _____ mg/hr   _____ ml/hr

16. Heparin is to be given at a rate of 1000 U/hr. If the drug is available as 10,000 U per 100 ml of fluid, how many ml/hr should be administered?

    _____ ml/hr

ANSWERS

Calculation of IV Fluids (pp. 127–133)

1. 19	23. 20	45. 21	67. 50
2. 100	24. 81	46. 75	68. 35
3. 31	25. 50	47. 125	69. 25
4. 125	26. 42	48. 21	70. 75
5. 75	27. 175	49. 30	71. 63
6. 13	28. 50	50. 10	72. 13
7. 125	29. 100	51. 13	73. 38
8. 13	30. 75	52. 19	74. 42
9. 83	31. 69	53. 5	75. 19
10. 50	32. 21	54. 21	76. 4
11. 38	33. 16	55. 10	77. 25
12. 58	34. 20	56. 4	78. 8
13. 100	35. 29	57. 44	
14. 31	36. 42	58. 63	
15. 25	37. 19	59. 20	
16. 33	38. 56	60. 21	
17. 42	39. 75	61. 6	
18. 24	40. 125	62. 50	
19. 25	41. 31	63. 19	
20. 83	42. 31	64. 13	
21. 21	43. 63	65. 100	
22. 21	44. 31	66. 50	

Titrations (pp. 137–139)

1. 8.3 mcg/kg/min
2. 2.5 mcg/kg/min
3. 2400 mcg/hr
   24 ml/hr
4a. 280 mg/dose
4b. 40 mg/hr
   40 ml/hr
5. 3000 mcg/hr
6. 25 ml/hr
7. 160 mcg/kg/hr
8. 750 mcg/min
   45000 mcg/hr
   38 ml/hr
9. 17.57 U/min
   53 ml/hr

10. 3.3 mcg/kg/min
11. 0.036 mcg/kg/min
    2.17 mcg/kg/hr
12. 10 ml/hr
13. 14.7 mcg/kg/min
14. 3 mcg/kg/min
15. 2.11 mg/min
    126.6 mg/hr
    32 ml/hr
16. 10 ml/hr

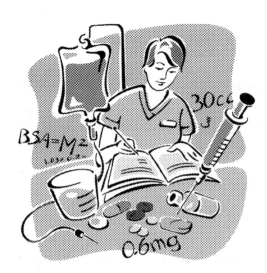

CHAPTER 12

Children's Dosage Calculations

When ordering drug dosages for children, physicians and advance practice nurses will probably use either a body surface area (BSA) or kilogram of body weight formula. These are accurate and correspond to drug manufacturers' information. To verify that an ordered dose is within safe limits, the nurse may use these formulas—as well as the traditional drug calculation rules based on age or weight.

Body Surface Area (BSA = M²)

This method of drug calculation is considered the most accurate, since it is based on a wider range of parameters. A body surface area nomogram, the child's height and weight, and the drug information in M² as listed by the drug manufacturer, are required to calculate this dosage.

Using the BSA nomogram, locate the child's height and weight. Draw a straight line between the two points. The intersection on the S.A. (M²) scale will be the estimated BSA (M²).

If the pediatric dosage in the drug manufacturers' literature is 10–50 mg/M²/day, use the lowest and highest ranges to calculate whether the dosage ordered is within the recommended range.

USING BODY SURFACE AREA (M²) TO DETERMINE CHILDREN'S DOSAGES

> **STEPS**
>
> **1.** Plot the height and weight on the nomogram. Connect the two points. Read the intersecting line on the S.A. scale to determine M².
>
> **2.** Multiply the lowest and highest dosage ranges by the M² to determine safe dosage range.

EXAMPLE: Child's height: 65 in   Weight: 95 lb
Dose ordered: 50 mg
Recommended range: 10–50 mg/M^2/day

Step 1: Plot height and weight on the nomogram. Connect the two points. The intersecting line on the S.A. scale is M^2 = 1.4.

Step 2: Multiply the lowest and highest dosage ranges by M^2 to determine safe dosage range.

lowest 10 $\times$ 1.4 = 14 mg

highest 50 $\times$ 1.4 = 70 mg

Conclusion: The 50 mg ordered is within the safe range of 14–70 mg.

EXAMPLE: Child's height: 110 cm   Weight: 30 kg
Dose ordered: 8 mg
Recommended range: 1.2 mg–6 mg/M^2/dose

Step 1: Plot height and weight on the nomogram. Connect the points. Read the S.A. scale to determine M^2.

M^2 = 0.98

Step 2: Multiply the lowest and highest dosage ranges by M^2 to determine safe dosage range.

lowest 1.2 mg $\times$ 0.98 = 1.18 mg

highest 6 mg $\times$ 0.98 = 5.88 mg

Conclusion: The 8 mg ordered is not within the safe range of 1.18–5.88 mg. Contact your prescriber.

Occasionally a prescriber may order a drug to be given in M^2.

EXAMPLE: Give Imuran 120 mg/M^2/daily po
Child's height: 80 cm   Weight: 10 kg

Step 1: Plot height and weight on the nomogram and connect the two points. The S.A. (M^2) = 0.48.

Step 2: Multiply the dose by the M^2.

120 $\times$ 0.48 = 57.6 mg.

Conclusion: 57.6 mg is the amount to be given.

EXAMPLE: Give Epinephrine 0.3 ml/M^2. The child's height is 42 in, and the weight is 30 lb.

Step 1: Plot height and weight on nomogram. Connect the two points. The BSA (M^2) = 0.62.

Step 2: Multiply the dose by M².

$$0.3 \text{ ml} \times 0.62 = 0.19 \text{ ml}$$

Answer: Give 0.19 ml.

Body Surface Area Using Adult Dosage

The BSA may also be used to determine a pediatric dose using the recommended adult dosage. The formula is:

$$\frac{\text{Child's BSA (M}^2)}{1.73 \text{ (M}^2)} = \times \text{ Adult dose} = \text{Child's dose}$$

EXAMPLE: Child's height: 31 in   Weight: 33 lb
Dose ordered: 3 mg
Adult dose: Valium 10 mg

Step 1: Plot height and weight on the nomogram and connect the two points. Determine the S.A.

$$(\text{M}^2) = 0.6$$

Step 2: Use the data in the formula.

$$\frac{0.6}{1.73} = 0.346 \times 10 \text{ (Adult dose)} = 3.46$$

Conclusion: Child's dose = 3.46. The dose ordered is a safe dose to administer.

EXAMPLE: Child's height: 30 in   Weight: 27 lb
Dose ordered: 150 mg
Adult dose: 500 mg

Step 1: Plot height and weight on the nomogram. Connect the points. The BSA (M²) = 0.54.

Step 2: Use formula $\frac{\text{BSA}}{1.73} \times$ Adult dose = Child's dose

$$\frac{0.54}{1.73} = 0.31 \times 500 = 155 \text{ mg}$$

Conclusion: Child's dose = 155 mg. The 150 mg ordered is a safe dose to give.

FIGURE 12.1 Nomogram for estimation of surface area, reprinted with permission from Behrman, R.E., Kliegman, R.M., and Ervin, A.M. Nelson Textbook of Pediatrics, 15th ed., W.B. Saunders Company, Philadelphia, PA 19105.

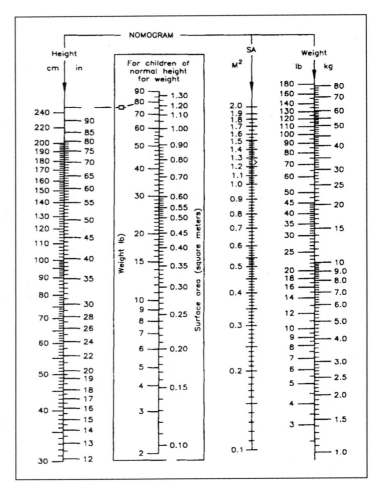

Plot height and weight. Connect the two points with a straight line. The intersection on the S.A. (M²) scale will be the estimated BSA (M²). If the child is average in height for weight, use weight alone and refer to the enclosed scale.

PRACTICE PROBLEMS—BODY SURFACE AREA

Solve:

1. Height: 53 in   Weight: 70 lb
Dose ordered: 0.5 g/M²   BSA _____
Give ____ g

2. Height: 20 in   Weight: 10 lb
Dose ordered: 150 mg/M²   BSA _____
Give ____ mg

3. Height: Average   Weight: 17 lb
Dose ordered: 50 mg daily
Recommended range: 60–90 mg/M²/day   BSA _____
Safe ____ Unsafe ____

4. Height: 90 cm   Weight: 15 kg
Dose ordered: 28 mg daily
Recommended range: 30–45 mg/M²/day   BSA _____
Safe _____ Unsafe _____

5. Height: 50 cm   Weight: 6 kg
Dose ordered: 180 mg/M²
Dose on hand: 100 mg/ml   BSA _____
Give _____ mg
Give _____ ml

6. Height: 85 cm   Weight: 40 lb
Dose ordered: 1.5 g/M²/qid
Dose on hand: 1000 mg/10 ml   BSA _____
Give _____ g
Give _____ ml

7. Epinephrine is ordered based on 0.3 ml/M²/dose. The dose available is labeled 1 mg/ml. The child is 25 in tall and weighs 26 lb. What is the BSA? How much would be given?   BSA _____
Give _____ ml

8. The recommended dose of Codeine for a child is 100 mg/M²/24 hours, given every four hours. A child who weighs 20 kg and is 80 cm tall would receive how much per dose?   BSA _____
Dose _____ mg

9. Keflin 1.5 g/M²/24 hours given qid is the recommended child's dose. A child whose BSA is 0.32 M² would receive how much for each dose?   _____ mg

10. Meperidine 175 mg/M²/24 hr, divided into six doses, is the recommended child's dose. A child whose BSA is 1.38 would receive how much each dose?   _____ mg

Body Surface Area Using Adult Dose

11. Height: 19 in   Weight: 8 lb
    Adult dose: 100 mg   BSA _____
                                          Child's Dose ____ mg

12. Height: 28 in   Weight: 22 lb
    Adult dose: 65 mg   BSA _____
                                          Child's dose ____ mg

13. Height: 65 cm   Weight: 7 kg
    Adult dose: 300 mg   BSA _____
                                          Child's dose ____ mg

14. Height: 100 cm   Weight: 25 kg
    Adult dose: 25 mg   BSA _____
                                          Child's dose ____ mg

15. Height: 30 in   Weight: 24 lb
    Adult dose: 10 mg   BSA _____
                                          Child's dose ____ mg

16. The adult dose of Morphine is 15 mg. A child with a BSA of 0.81 M^2 would receive how much?   ____ mg

17. Decadron 4 mg is an adult dose. A child with a BSA of 0.55 M^2 would receive how much?   ____ mg

18a. The adult dose of Atropine is 0.4 mg. How much would a child with a BSA of 0.34 M^2 receive?   ____ mg

18b. Atropine is available in a vial labeled $\frac{1}{150}$ gr per 0.5 ml. Based on the dose computed above, how much would you give? _____ ml

19a. Aminophyllin 250 mg is an adult dose. A child with a BSA of 0.59 M² would receive what dose? _____ mg

19b. Aminophyllin is available in vials labeled 250 mg/ml. Based on the dose computed above, how much would you give? _____ ml

20. Chloral Hydrate 750 mg is an adult dose. How much would a child with a BSA of 1.6 M² receive? _____ mg

---

Kilogram of Body Weight

This method of calculating pediatric dosages is the most commonly used method, and most drug manufacturers' information gives the pediatric dosage in this form. To calculate this dosage, the nurse needs the child's weight in kg and the recommended dosage as described by the drug manufacturer.

STEPS

1. Convert weight to kg if necessary (2.2 lb = 1 kg).
2. Multiply recommended dose by kg.

EXAMPLE: A child weighing 35 lb is ordered Atropine 0.15 mg IM on call to OR. To verify the safety of this dosage, note that the drug manufacturer's recommended dose is 0.01 mg/kg/dose.

Step 1: Convert 35 lb to kg.

$$\frac{2.2}{1} = \frac{35}{X}$$

2.2 X = 35

X = 15.9

Step 2: Multiply 15.9 kg × recommended dose.

0.01 × 15.9 = 0.159 mg

Conclusion: The dosage ordered (0.15 mg) is a safe dose to administer.

EXAMPLE: The order reads, "Hydroxyzine 12.5 mg IM now." The recommended dose is 1 mg/kg. If the child weighs 25 lb, would this be an appropriate dose to give?

Step 1: Convert lb to kg.

$$\frac{2.2\ lb}{kg} = \frac{25}{X}$$

$$2.2X = 25$$
$$X = \frac{25}{2.2}$$
$$X = 11.36\ kg$$

Step 2: Multiply kg by the recommended dose.

$$11.36\ kg \times 1\ mg = 11.36\ mg$$

Conclusion: Child's dose = 11.36 mg. The dose ordered (12.5 mg) is an appropriate dose to administer.

PRACTICE PROBLEMS—KILOGRAM OF BODY WEIGHT

Solve:

1. Weight 8.8 lb
   Dose ordered: 30 mg po bid
   Dose recommended: 15 mg/kg/24 hr

   Safe _____
   Unsafe _____
   _____ mg/24 hr

2. Weight: 3.2 kg
   Dose ordered: 40 mg po qid
   Dose recommended: 50–100 mg/kg/24 hours

   Safe _____
   Unsafe _____
   _____ mg/qid

3. Weight: 72 lb
   Dose ordered: Hydroxyzine 50 mg IM
   Dose recommended: 1.1 mg/kg

   Safe _____
   Unsafe _____
   _____ mg/dose

4. Weight: 16 lb
   Dose ordered: Paregoric 2 ml
   Dose recommended: 0.25–0.5 ml/kg/dose

   Safe _____
   Unsafe _____
   _____ ml/dose

5. Weight: 21.8 kg
   Dose ordered: Kanamycin 200 mg q8h
   Dose recommended: 15 mg/kg/day   Safe _____
                                                       Unsafe _____
                                                       _____ mg/day

6. Aspirin 300 mg is ordered for a child weighing 40 lb. The recommended amount for children is 65 mg/kg/24 hr, divided into six doses. Aspirin is available in tablets labeled 5 gr each. Would this order be safe,
   and if not, what would be a safe dose?   Safe _____
                                                          Unsafe _____
                                                          _____ mg

7. Tofranil 1.5 mg/kg/24 hr, divided into four doses, is the recommended dose for a child. How much should a child weighing 80 lb
   receive?   _____ mg

8a. Garamycn 3 mg/kg/24 hr, divided into three doses, is the rec-
    ommended dose for a child. How much would a child weighing
    20 kg receive?
    _____ mg

8b. The drug is available labeled Garamycin 40 mg/ml. Based on the
    dose computed above, how much would you give?   _____ ml

9. The recommended child's dose of Ampicillin is 50–100 mg/kg/24
   hr, divided into four doses. An acceptable range for a child weighing 18 lb would be?
                                                          _____ mg/day
                                                          _____ mg/dose

10. Promethazine 1 mg/kg/24 hr, divided into six doses, is the rec-
    ommended child's dose. A child weighing 28 lb would receive
    how much for each dose?   _____ mg

Traditional Rules Using Adult Dosage

The following formulas may be used to verify that an ordered dosage is within safe limits; however, these are less accurate than the previously discussed methods. The dosage calculated by any of these rules may range ±10 and still be considered within a safe range. In the event the dosage ordered exceeds 10 percent of what the nurse calculates as safe, the prescriber must be contacted to discuss the dosage ordered.

FRIED'S RULE (AGE IN MONTHS)

$$\text{Infant's dosage} = \frac{\text{Age in months}}{150} \times \text{Adult dosage}$$

EXAMPLE: If the adult dosage of a drug is 100 mg, what would be a safe dosage for a 9-month-old child?

$$\frac{9}{150} \times 100 = \frac{900}{150} = 6 \text{ mg}$$

YOUNG'S RULE (AGE IN YEARS)

$$\text{Child's dosage} = \frac{\text{Age of child in years}}{\text{Age of child plus 12}} \times \text{Adult dosage}$$

EXAMPLE: Usual adult dosage of Atropine is $\frac{1}{150}$ gr. What is a safe dosage for a 6-year-old child?

$$\frac{6}{6 + 12} \times \frac{1}{150} = \frac{\overset{1}{\cancel{6}}}{18} \times \frac{1}{\underset{25}{\cancel{150}}} = \frac{1}{450} \text{ gr}$$

CLARK'S RULE (WEIGHT)

$$\text{Child's dosage} = \frac{\text{Weight in pounds}}{150} \times \text{Adult dosage}$$

EXAMPLE: An adult dose of Ampicillin is 500 mg. How many mg should a child weighing 48 lb receive?

$$\frac{48}{\underset{3}{\cancel{150}}} \times \overset{10}{\cancel{500}} = \frac{480}{3} = 160 \text{ mg}$$

PRACTICE PROBLEMS—DOSAGE USING TRADITIONAL RULES

Use the appropriate traditional rule (Fried's, Young's, or Clark's) to calculate the child's dose.

	Adult Dosage	Age/Weight Information	Child Dosage
1.	Aldactone 25 mg	5 years	_____ mg
2.	Seconal 200 mg	99 lb	_____ mg

	Adult Dosage	Age/Weight Information	Child Dosage
3.	Phenergan 25 mg	7 years	_____ mg
4.	Valium 10 mg	6 months	_____ mg
5.	Regitine 5 mg	16 lb	_____ mg

6. The usual adult dosage of Tofranil is 50 mg. What would be a safe dosage for a 6-year-old child?

7. The adult dosage of Valium is 10 mg. What is a safe dosage for a 25-lb child?

8. The usual adult dosage of Robinul is $\frac{1}{300}$ gr. How much should a 6-month-old receive?

9. Talwin 75 mg is an adult dosage. What would be a safe dosage for a 13-year-old child?

10. Dalmane 30 mg is an adult dosage. What is a safe dosage for a 70-lb child?

11. The usual adult dosage of ASA is 600 mg. How much would be given to a 4-year-old child?

12. Milk of Magnesia 30 ml is the usual adult dosage. What would be a safe amount to give a 16-month-old child?

ANSWERS

Body Surface Area (pp. 144–147)

1. BSA 1.1
0.55 g
2. BSA 0.27
40.5 mg
3. BSA 0.39
Unsafe
4. BSA 0.62
Safe
5. BSA 0.31
55.8 mg
0.56 ml

6. BSA 0.68
0.3 g
3 ml
7. BSA 0.49
0.15 ml
8. BSA 0.7
12 mg
9. 120 mg
10. 40.25 mg

Body Surface Area Using Adult Dose (pp. 146–147)

11. BSA 0.23
    13.2 mg
12. BSA 0.46
    17.23 mg
13. BSA 0.37
    64.2 mg

14. BSA 0.88
    12.7 mg
15. BSA 0.5
    2.9 mg
16. 7 mg
17. 1.27 mg

18a. 0.08 mg
18b. 0.1 ml
19. 85 mg
    0.34 ml
20. 694 mg

Kilogram of Body Weight (pp. 148–149)

1. Safe
   60 mg/24 hr
2. Safe
   40–80 mg/24 hr
3. Unsafe
   36 mg/dose

4. Safe
   1.8–3.6 ml/dose
5. Unsafe
   327 mg/day
6. Unsafe
   195 mg

7. 13.65 mg
8. 20 mg
   0.5 ml
9. 409–818 mg/day
   102–205 mg/dose
10. 2.12 mg

Dosage Using Traditional Rules (pp. 150–151)

1. 7.35 mg

2. 132 mg

3. 9.2 mg

4. 0.4 mg

5. 0.53 mg

6. 16.7 mg

7. 1.67 mg

8. $\frac{1}{7500}$ gr

9. 39 mg

10. 14 mg

11. 150 mg

12. 3.2 ml

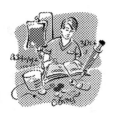

UNIT 3

Comprehensive Test

Calculate the following oral, parenteral, IV rate, and children's dosage problems:

1. Dose ordered: Paregoric 3 ii po
    Dose on hand: Paregoric liquid

    Give _____ ml

2. Dose ordered: Tetracycline 1 g po
    Dose on hand: Tetracycline 500 mg cap

    Give _____ cap

3. Dose ordered: Allopurinol 250 mg po
    Dose on hand: Allopurinol 100 mg

    Give _____ tab

4. Dose ordered: Atenolol 75 mg po
    Dose on hand: Atenolol 25 mg tab

    Give _____ tab

5. Dose ordered: Ergotamine 0.6 mg SL
    Dose on hand: Ergotamine 0.2 mg tab

    Give _____ tab

6. Dose ordered: Ciprofloxacin 0.5 g po
    Dose on hand: Ciprofloxacin 250 mg cap

    Give _____ cap

7. Dose ordered: Tagamet 300 mg po
   Dose on hand: Tagamet 0.6 g tablet   Give ＿＿ tab

8. Dose ordered: Valium 5 mg po
   Dose on hand: Valium 2.5 mg tablet   Give ＿＿ tab

9. Dose ordered: Edecrin 50 mg po
   Dose on hand: Edecrin $\frac{3}{4}$ gr tablet   Give ＿＿ tab

10. Dose ordered: Lanoxin 0.025 mg po
    Dose on hand: Lanoxin 0.05 mg/5 ml   Give ＿＿ ml

11. Give Acetaminophen 325 mg from tablets labeled Acetaminophen
    5 gr.   ＿＿ tab

12. The order reads Indomethacin 50 mg po. The drug is available labeled Indomethacin 25 mg/5 ml.   ＿＿ ml

13. Give Cloxacillin 1 g from capsules labeled Cloxacillin 250 mg.
                                                         ＿＿ cap

14. Give Dipyridamole 0.1 g from tablets labeled Dipyridamole 50 mg.   ＿＿ tab

15. Give Etodolac 600 mg po from capsules labeled Etodolac 300 mg.
                                                         ＿＿ cap

16. The order reads Fosinopril 40 mg. The drug is available as tablets labeled Fosinopril 10 mg.   ＿＿ tab

17. Give Ritalin 10 mg po from tablets labeled Ritalin 2.5 mg.
                                                         ＿＿ tab

18. Give Minocin 200 mg po from capsules labeled 0.1 g.

_____ cap

19. The order reads Serax 15 mg. The drug is available labeled Serax $\frac{1}{2}$ gr.   _____ tab

20. Give Lithium 0.3 g from capsules labeled Lithium 300 mg.

_____ cap

21. The order reads Meclofenamate 150 mg. The drug is available labeled Meclofenamate 50 mg.   _____ cap

22. Give Dilantin 90 mg from a bottle labeled Dilantin 30 mg/5 ml.

_____ ml

23. Give Kaon Elixir 20 mEq from the drug labeled Kaon Elixir 10 mEq/5 ml.   _____ ml

24. Give Mysoline 0.125 g from tablets labeled 250 mg.   _____ tab

25. Give Mellaril 25 mg from tablets labeled Mellaril $\frac{1}{6}$ gr.   _____ tab

26. Give Dalgan 2.5 mg IV. It is available as 10 mg per ml.   _____ ml

27. The written order is Pentobarbital 100 mg. The drug is available as 50 mg per ml.   _____ ml

28. The order is for Perphenazine 10 mg. It is in an ampule labeled 5 mg per ml.   _____ ml

29. Give Phenobarbital Sodium 65 mg IM. The drug is available as 130 mg per ml.   _____ ml

30. Phenytoin Sodium 100 mg IV is ordered. It is in a vial labeled 50 mg per ml.   _____ ml

31. Add Potassium Chloride 20 mEq to an IV solution. The drug is available as 40 mEq per 20 ml.   _____ ml

32. A drug order is for Amikacin 150 mg q8hr IM. The drug is available as 250 mg/ml.   _____ ml

33. Give Atropine 0.75 mg IV. The drug is available in a vial labeled 0.5 mg/ml.   _____ ml

34. Biperidin 2 mg IM is ordered. The vial label reads 1 ml = 5 mg.   _____ ml

35. Give Benadryl 12.5 mg IV. The vial is labeled 1 ml = 50 mg.   _____ ml

36. A drug order is for Cephradin 500 mg IM. The label reads each ml = 200 mg.   _____ ml

37. Give Cefazolin 275 mg IM. When 2.0 ml of sterile diluent is added to the 500 mg vial, each ml = 225 mg.   Give _____ ml

38. A drug order is for Erythromycin 500 mg IV q6hr. When 20 ml of diluent are added to the 1 g vial, each cc = 50 mg.
                                                                         Give _____ cc

39. Methotrexate 10 mg IV is ordered. When diluted with 20 ml of diluent, the vial contains 0.02 g per ml. Give _____ ml

40. Cetazidime 560 mg IV is available in a 1 g vial. When diluted with 3 ml sterile water, each ml = 280 mg. Give _____ ml

41. Give Ampicillin Sodium 500 mg IV q6hr. The drug is available in a 1 g vial. When the drug is diluted with 10 ml sterile water each ml = 50 mg. Give _____ ml

Calculate the dosages for the following two pre-ops.

42. Give Dilaudid 1 mg
   Versed 1 mg   > IM on call to OR
   Robinul 0.2 mg

   On hand: Dilaudid 2 mg/ml, Versed 2 mg/2 ml,
       Robinul 0.2 mg/ml

   Dilaudid _____ ml, Versed _____ ml, Robinul _____ ml

43. Give Demerol 35 mg and Benadryl 12.5 mg IM. On hand is Demerol 50 mg/ml and Benadryl 50 mg/ml.
   Demerol _____ ml
   Benadryl _____ ml

44. Give Heparin 2500 U sub-q from a vial labeled 5000 U per cc. _____ cc

45. Give Procaine Penicillin 600,000 U IM from a vial labeled 300,000 U per ml. _____ ml

46. Infuse 200 ml of $D_5 \frac{1}{4}$ NS over 3 hr. Using a drop factor of 10, you would regulate the flow rate at _____ gtt/min.

47. Infuse 2400 ml of Ringer's Lactate solution over 8 hr. Using a microdrip administration set, regulate the flow rate at _____ gtt/min.

48. Use a standard IV administration set and infuse 400 ml of fluid over 6 hr. _____ gtt/min

49. A unit of whole blood (500 ml) running over 4 hr should be regulated at _____ gtt/min

50. Infuse 225 ml of $\frac{1}{2}$ strength saline over 3 hr. Use a microdrip administration set. _____ gtt/min

51. Infuse 500 ml of fluid over 8 hr. Using an administration set with a drop factor of 20, regulate the flow rate at _____ gtt/min.

52. Administer 2400 ml of $D_5 \frac{1}{2}$ NS over 12 hr. Using a drop factor of 10, regulate the flow rate at _____ gtt/min.

53. Administer 900 ml of fluid over 8 hr. Using a drop factor of 60, regulate the flow rate at _____ gtt/min.

54. Infuse 300 ml of $D_5 \frac{1}{4}$ NS over 6 hr. Using a standard IV administration set, regulate the flow rate at _____ gtt/min.

55. Infuse 1200 ml Normosol over 6 hr. Use a drop factor of 10, regulate the flow rate at _____ gtt/min.

Calculate the following rates:

	Amount of Fluid	Time	IV Set Drop Factor	Gtt/Min
56.	600 ml	8 hr	10	_____
57.	500 ml	6 hr	15	_____
58.	250 ml	4 hr	20	_____
59.	125 ml	1 hr	60	_____

	Amount of Fluid	Time	IV Set Drop Factor	Gtt/Min
60.	225 ml	1 hr	15	_____
61.	1500 ml	12 hr	60	_____
62.	375 ml	4 hr	60	_____
63.	800 ml	6 hr	10	_____
64.	85 ml	1 hr	60	_____
65.	1000 ml	8 hr	20	_____
66.	1200 ml	24 hr	10	_____
67.	250 ml	4 hr	60	_____
68.	225 ml	3 hr	60	_____
69.	125 ml	1 hr	20	_____
70.	46 ml	1 hr	60	_____

71. The usual adult dosage of Acetaminophen is 325 mg. What dosage would be appropriate for a 6-year-old child? (Young's Rule)
_____ mg

72. Keflex 500 mg is the usual adult dosage. What is the dosage for a 10-year-old child? (Young's Rule) _____ mg

73. The adult dosage of Chloromycetin is 100 mg. How much should a 6-month-old receive? (Fried's Rule) _____ mg

74. Chlorothiazide 1 g is the usual adult dosage. How much should an 18-month-old receive? (Fried's Rule) _____ mg

75. The usual adult dosage of Edecrin is 50 mg. What would a 38-lb child's dosage be? (Clark's Rule) _____ mg

76. Aminophyllin 500 mg is a usual adult dose. What dose is recommended for a child weighing 46 lb? (Clark's Rule)

_____ mg

77. Ritalin 15 mg/M²/dose is recommended. How much would a child who weighs 85 lb and is 47 in tall receive?

BSA _____

_____ mg

78. Phenylephrine 3 mg/M²/dose is recommended. How much would a child whose BSA = 0.92 receive? _____ mg

79. Phenylephrine 3 mg IM is ordered. The drug is available in an ampule labeled 10 mg/ml. How much should be given?

_____ ml

80. Erythromycin 200 mg po is ordered for a child weighing 5 kg. The recommended dose is 30–50 mg/kg. Would the dose ordered be within a safe range for administration? Safe _____

Unsafe _____

81. Phenytoin 50 mg twice a day is ordered for a child weighing 32 lb. The recommended dose is 3–8 mg/kg/24 hr. Would the dose ordered be within a safe range for administration?

Safe _____

Unsafe _____

82. Chloral Hydrate 1.5 g/M²/24 hr is recommended. How much would a child who weighs 18 lb and is 28 in tall receive?

BSA _____

_____ g

83. Atropine 0.4 mg is the usual adult dosage. How much should a child who weighs 7 kg and is 65 cm long receive?   BSA _____

_____ mg

84. Atropine is available in ampules labeled 0.4 mg/0.5 ml. To give Atropine 0.09 mg, how much would you give?   _____ ml

85. Morphine Sulfate 10 mg is an adult dose. How much should a child who weighs 18 lb and is 26 in long receive?   BSA _____

_____ mg

86. Meperidine 100 mg is an adult dose. How much would a child weighing 23 kg and measuring 116 cm receive?   BSA _____

_____ mg

87. Reserpine 0.02 mg/kg/day is recommended. How much should a child who weighs 55 lb receive?   _____ mg

88. Theophyllin 20 mg/kg/24 hr given po every six hours is recommended. How much would a child who weighs 42 lb receive per dose?   _____ mg

89. Ticarcillin 200 mg/kg/24 hr given IV every four hours is recommended. How much would a child who weighs 26 kg receive per dose?   _____ mg

90. Gentamycin 3 mg/kg/24 hr given every eight hours is recommended. How much would a child who weighs 24 kg receive per dose?   _____ mg

91. Tofranil 1.5 mg/kg/24 hr divided into four doses is recommended. How much would a child weighing 52 lb receive per dose?   _____ mg

92. A patient is receiving a drug which has been titrated at 42 ml/hr. The drug is mixed as 500 mg/500 ml of fluid. The patient weighs 70 kg. How many mcg/kg/min is the patient receiving?

_____ mcg/kg/min

93. Give Dopamine at a rate of 8 ml/hr to a patient who weighs 132 lb. The drug is mixed as 400 mg/500 ml of fluid. How many mcg/kg/hr is the patient receiving?

_____ mcg/kg/hr

94. Heparin is to be given at a rate of 1500 U/hr IV. If the drug is available as 10,000 U per 100 ml of fluid, how many ml/hr should be administered?

_____ ml/hr

95. You are to infuse Nipride 3 mcg/kg/min from a solution of 50 mg in 250 ml D_5 W. The patient weighs 166 lb. How many mcg/min will be given? What will be the infusion pump rate?

_____ mcg/min   _____ ml/hr

96. Amrinone 250 mg in 500 ml of fluid is to infuse at 5 mcg/kg/min for a patient weighing 96 kg. How many mcg/hr will be given? At what rate should the infusion pump be set?

_____ mcg/hr   _____ ml/hr

97. Add 1 g of medication to 500 ml of fluid and infuse at a rate of 1 mg per minute. What will be the infusion pump rate?

_____ ml/hr

98. Infuse Nitroprusside 1.5 mcg/kg/min to a patient weighing 198 lb. The solution is mixed 50 mg in 250 ml D_5 W. How many mcg/min will be given, and what will the infusion rate be?

_____ mcg/min   _____ ml/hr

99. Give Isuprel 0.084 mcg/kg/min from a solution mixed 2 mg per 500 ml to a patient weighing 130 lb. How many mcg/min will be given? How many mcg/hr? What will be the infusion pump rate?   _____ mcg/min   _____ mcg/hr   _____ ml/hr

100. A patient weighing 62 kg is receiving a drug which has been titrated for effect at 12 ml/hr. The drug is mixed 200 mg/250 ml of fluid. How many mcg/kg/min is the patient receiving?

_____ mcg/kg/min

ANSWERS

Unit 3: Comprehensive Test (pp. 153–162)

1. 10 ml	**24.** $\frac{1}{2}$ tab	**45.** 2 ml
2. 2 cap	**25.** $2\frac{1}{2}$ tab	**46.** 11
3. $2\frac{1}{2}$ tab	**26.** 0.25 ml	**47.** 300
4. 3 tab	**27.** 2 ml	**48.** 17
5. 3 tab	**28.** 2 ml	**49.** 20
6. 2 cap	**29.** 0.5 ml	**50.** 75
7. $\frac{1}{2}$ tab	**30.** 2 ml	**51.** 21
8. 2 tab	**31.** 10 ml	**52.** 33
9. 1 tab	**32.** 0.6 ml	**53.** 113
10. 2.5 ml	**33.** 1.5 ml	**54.** 13
11. 1 tab	**34.** 0.4 ml	**55.** 33
12. 10 ml	**35.** 0.25 ml	**56.** 13
13. 4 cap	**36.** 2.5 ml	**57.** 21
14. 2 tab	**37.** 1.22 ml	**58.** 21
15. 2 cap	**38.** 10 cc	**59.** 125
16. 4 tab	**39.** 0.5 ml	**60.** 56
17. 4 tab	**40.** 2 ml	**61.** 125
18. 2 cap	**41.** 10 ml	**62.** 94
19. $\frac{1}{2}$ tab	**42.** Dilaudid 0.5 ml	**63.** 22
20. 1 cap	Versed 1 ml	**64.** 85
21. 3 cap	Robinul 1 ml	**65.** 42
22. 15 ml	**43.** Demerol 0.7 ml	**66.** 8
23. 10 ml	Benadryl 0.25 ml	**67.** 63
	44. 0.5 cc	

68. 75

69. 42

70. 46

71. 108 mg

72. 227 mg

73. 4 mg

74. 120 mg

75. 13 mg

76. 155 mg

77. BSA 1.16
17.4 mg

78. 2.76 mg

79. 0.3 ml

80. Safe
150–250 mg

81. Safe
43.6–116.3 mg

82. BSA 0.41
0.615 g

83. BSA 0.37
0.085 mg

84. 0.11 ml

85. BSA 0.4
2.3 mg

86. BSA 0.85
50 mg

87. 0.5 mg

88. 95.45 mg

89. 866.6 mg

90. 24 mg

91. 8.86 mg

92. 10
mcg/kg/min

93. 106.67
mcg/kg/hr

94. 15 ml

95. 226.35 mcg/min
68 ml/hr

96. 28,800 mcg/hr
58 ml/hr

97. 30 ml/hr

98. 135 mcg/min
41 ml/hr

99. 4.96 mcg/min
297.6 mcg/hr
74 ml/hr

100. 2.58
mcg/kg/min

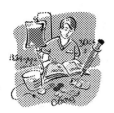

Comprehensive Exam

1. 34°C = _____ °F

2. 117°F = _____ °C

3. 324 ml = _____ L

4. 16.5 L = _____ cc

5. 10.5 kl = _____ L

6. 16.7 kg = _____ g

7. 3.2 g = _____ mcg

8. 0.02 mg = _____ mcg

9. 39.4 g = _____ kg

10. 164 ml = _____ kl

11. 17.3 ml = _____ cc

12. 14,000 mcg = _____ g

13. 34 in. = _____ cm

14. 129 cm = _____ in

15. 120 ml = _____ ʒ = _____ ʒ

16. 35 m$_x$ = _____ cc

17. 15 ml = _____ ʒ = _____ Tbsp

18. 65 kg = _____ lb

19. 250 ml = ____ pt = ____ ʒ

20. 0.01 mg = ____ gr

21. 14.5 L = ____ ml = ____ qt

22. 0.6 mg = ____ gr

23. 250 mg = ____ gr = ____ g

24. 0.5 ml = ____ gtt

25. 100 kg = ____ lb = ____ mg

26. $\frac{1}{500}$ gr = ____ mg

27. 3 pt = ____ qt

28. 45 m_x = ____ ml

29. ʒ $\overline{\text{iii}}$ = ____ ml

30. 4 Tbsp = ____ ml

31. 4 qt = ____ gal

32. $\frac{1}{20}$ gr = ____ mg

33. gr vii$\overline{\text{ss}}$ ____ mg = ____ g

34. 2 glasses = ____ ml

35. 1 qt = ____ ml

36. ʒ vi = ____ glass

37. 8 m_x = ____ ml

38. ʒii$\overline{\text{ss}}$ = ____ ml

39. $\frac{1}{5}$ gr = ____ mg = ____ g

40. $\frac{1}{120}$ gr = ____ mg

41. 5 teacups = ____ ml

42. i$\overline{\text{ss}}$ gal = ____ ml

43. 16 m_x = ____ ml

44. ʒ $\overline{\text{x}}$ = ____ ml

45. 4 qt = _____ gal

48. 3̄viii = _____ tsp

46. 10 Tbsp = _____ ml

49. 6 pt = _____ qt

47. gr vi = _____ g = _____ mg

50. gr iii = _____ mg

51. Give Acyclovir 250 mg. The drug is available labeled Acyclovir 200 mg/5 ml.   Give _____ ml

52. The order reads Busulfan 8 mg po. The drug is labeled Busulfan 2 mg per tablet.   Give _____ tab

53. Give Cefaclor 250 mg. Cefaclor is labeled 125 mg/5 ml.
                                                    Give _____ ml

54. The order reads Keflex 250 mg po. The drug is available Keflex 125 mg/5 ml.   Give _____ ml

55. Chlordiazepoxide 20 mg po is ordered. The drug is available as 10 mg capsules.   Give _____ cap

56. Give Hydrochlorothiazide 25 mg qod from tablets labeled 50 mg.
                                                    Give _____ tab

57. Give Cleocin 0.075 g from a bottle labeled 75 mg/5 ml.
                                                    Give _____ ml

58. The order reads Codeine $\frac{1}{4}$ gr. You have Codeine 30 mg tabs.
                                                    Give _____ tab

59. Give Thorazine 25 mg po. The drug is available labeled Thorazine 10 mg/5 ml.   Give _____ ml

60. Give Periactin 2 mg from drug labeled Periactin 2 mg/5 ml. How many tsp should be given?   Give _____ tsp

61. Give Valium 2.5 mg from tablets labeled Valium 5 mg.
                                                          Give _____ tab

62. Give Declomycin 0.3 g q12h from capsules labeled Declomycin 150 mg.   Give _____ cap

63. Give Elixir Benadryl 10 mg from a bottle labeled Elixir Benadryl 12.5 mg/5 ml.   Give _____ ml

64. Give Lanoxin 0.035 mg from a bottle labeled Lanoxin 0.25 mg/ 5 ml.   Give _____ ml

65. The order reads Lasix 10 mg po. The available drug is labeled Lasix 40 mg/5 ml.   Give _____ ml

66. Give Clozapine 125 mg from tablets labeled Clozapine 25 mg.
                                                          Give _____ tab

67. Give TheoDur 160 mg from a bottle labeled TheoDur 80 mg/15 ml.
                                                          Give _____ ml

68. Give Danazol 400 mg po from Danazol 200 mg capsules.
                                                          Give _____ cap

69. The order reads Vistaril 10 mg po qid. The drug is available labeled Vistaril 25 mg/5 ml.   Give _____ ml

70. Give Tofranil 25 mg from a solution labeled Tofranil 12.5 mg/ml.   Give _____ ml

71. The order reads Doxepin 25 mg. The drug is available as Doxepin 10 mg/ml.   Give _____ ml

72. Give Mycostatin 150,000 U from a solution labeled Mycostatin 100,000 U/ml.   Give _____ ml

73. Give V-Cillin K 125 mg po from a bottle labeled 250 mg per 5 ml.   Give _____ ml

74. Give Mysoline 0.1 g po from a bottle labeled Mysoline 250 mg/5 ml.   Give _____ ml

75. Give Methadone 7.5 mg po from a bottle labeled 5 mg per 5 ml.   Give _____ ml

76. Give Procainamide HC1 200 mg IV. The drug is available as 0.5 g per ml.   Give _____ ml

77. Prochlorperazine 10 mg IM is ordered. It is in a vial labeled 5 mg per ml.   Give _____ ml

78. The written order is Promazine HC1 12.5 mg IM. It is available as 0.025 g per ml.   Give _____ ml

79. Give Deferoxamine 1 g q12h. The drug is in a vial labeled 500 mg/2 ml. Give _____ ml

80. Propranolol 3 mg IV is ordered. It is available as 1 mg per ml. Give _____ ml

81. Give Quinidine 400 mg IM q12h. The vial on hand is 80 mg per ml. Give _____ ml

82. The order reads Glycopyrrolate 200 mcg IM. The drug is available as 0.2 mg/ml. Give _____ ml

83. Iron Dextran 125 mg IM is ordered. It is in a vial labeled as 50 mg/ml. Give _____ ml

84. Give Terbutaline Sulfate 250 mcg sub-q. It is available as 1 mg per ml. Give _____ m_x

85. The order is Thiothixene 4 mg IM bid. The vial is labeled 5 mg/ml. Give _____ ml

86. Ergocalciferol 10,000 U/day IM is ordered. The drug is available as 50,000 U/ml. Give _____ ml

87. Give Tobramycin 100 mg IV qid. It is available as 40 mg per ml. Give _____ ml

88. Give Chlordiazepoxide 25 mg IV. When the 50 mg vial is diluted with 5 ml of sterile diluent, each ml = 5 mg. Give _____ ml

89. Amikacin Sulfate 1 g IV is ordered. The 500 mg vial is diluted with 10 ml of sterile diluent so that each ml = 50 mg.

Give _____ ml

90. Ampicillin 125 mg IV is ordered. After the 500 mg vial is diluted with 5 ml of sterile water, each ml = 100 mg.   Give _____ ml

91. Methergine 100 mcg q12h IV is ordered. It is available as 0.2 mg/ml.   Give _____ ml

92. Mechlorethamine 7.5 mg IV is ordered. How much should be given if every 1 ml = 2 mg?   _____ ml

93. Methicillin 500 mg IM q6h is ordered. How much is given when the vial is labeled 1 g/2 ml?   _____ ml

94. Chlorthiazide 750 mg IV is ordered. How much is administered when each 2 ml = 500 mg?   _____ ml

95. Bleomycin 2 U IM is ordered. How much must be given when each 1 ml = 5 U?   _____ ml

96. Give the following pre-op:

Dilaudid 1.5 mg
               > IM
Robinul 0.2 mg

Dilaudid is available as 2 mg/ml
Robinul is available as 0.4 mg/2 ml

Dilaudid _____ ml   Robinul _____ ml

97. Give Heparin 2000 U sub-q from a vial labeled 10,000 U per ml.

Give _____ ml

Calculate the following gtt/min:

	Amount	Time	IV Set Drop Factor	Gtt/Min
98.	60 ml	1 hr	60	_____
99.	200 ml	3 hr	15	_____
100.	1200 ml	10 hr	20	_____
101.	600 ml	5 hr	10	_____
102.	480 ml	8 hr	60	_____
103.	1800 ml	12 hr	15	_____
104.	500 ml	6 hr	20	_____
105.	36 ml	1 hr	60	_____
106.	125 ml	2 hr	15	_____
107.	50 ml	$1\frac{1}{2}$ hr	10	_____
108.	800 ml	4 hr	15	_____
109.	75 ml	1 hr	60	_____
110.	1400 ml	8 hr	20	_____

	Amount	Time	IV Set Drop Factor	Gtt/Min
111.	120 ml	2 hr	10	____
112.	55 ml	1 hr	15	____

113. Infuse D_5 W 1000 ml over 6 hr. Using a standard IV administration set, regulate the rate at ____ gtt/min.

114. Infuse 150 ml of Hyperalimentation fluid over 2 hr. Use a microdrip administration set and regulate the rate at ____ gtt/min.

115. The order reads Ionosol MB 800 ml to infuse over 8 hr. Using a microdrip administration set, regulate the rate of ____ gtt/min.

116. Infuse $D_5 \frac{1}{2}$ NS 600 ml over 8 hr. Use a standard IV administration set and regulate the rate at ____ gtt/min.

117. Administer Human Plasma 250 ml over 3 hr. Use a blood administration IV set and regulate the rate at ____ gtt/min.

118. The order reads: $D_5 \frac{1}{4}$ NS 500 ml to infuse at 35 ml/hr. Using an IV set with a drop factor of 60, you would regulate the rate at ____ gtt/min.

119. Give Ringer's Lactate 500 ml over 4 hr. Using a standard IV administration set, regulate the rate at ____ gtt/min.

120. Infuse Dextran 6 percent 250 ml over 4 hr. Using a blood administration set, regulate the rate at ____ gtt/min.

121. Infuse D_{10} W 1000 ml over 12 hr. Use standard IV administration set and regulate the rate at _____ gtt/min.

122. Infuse $D_5 \frac{1}{2}$ NS 500 ml over 6 hr. Using a microdrip administration set, regulate the rate at _____ gtt/min.

Use the appropriate traditional rule (Young, Fried, Clark) to solve the following seven children's dosage problems.

	Adult Dosage	Age/Weight	Child's Dosage
123.	0.25 mg	14 lb	_____ mg
124.	0.26 g	4 years	_____ g
125.	$\frac{1}{6}$ gr	18 months	_____ gr
126.	180 mg	62 lb	_____ mg
127.	130 mg	12 years	_____ mg
128.	$\frac{1}{100}$ gr	3 months	_____ gr
129.	300,000 U	5 years	_____ U

130. If the adult dose of a drug is 20 mEq, how much would be appropriate for a child who has a BSA of 0.52 M^2? _____ mEq

131. Robinul 0.2 mg is an adult dose. How much would be acceptable for a child who weighs 24 lb and measures 85 cm long?

BSA _____

_____ mg

132. A common adult dosage of Lasix is 40 mg. How much would be safe for a child weighing 16 lb and measuring 28 in long?

BSA ____

____ mg

133. Penicillin G 600,000 U is an adult dose. How much would a child who weighs 31 lb and measures 100 cm long receive? BSA ____

____ U

134. Aldactone 25 mg is an adult dose. How much should a 1-year-old child whose BSA = 0.36 receive?

____ mg

135. Nafcillin 250 mg is an adult dose. A 10 lb infant who is 64 cm long would receive how much?

BSA ____

____ mg

136. The usual adult dose of Cleocin is 150 mg. A child weighing 44 lb and who is of normal height for his weight would receive how much?

BSA ____

____ mg

137. Hydroxyzine 60 mg/M²/24 hr given po in four doses is recommended. How much should a child who weighs 30 lb and measures 34 in long receive? BSA ____

____ mg

138. Paraldehyde 6 mg/M²/dose is recommended. How much should a child weighing 50 kg and measuring 146 cm receive?

BSA ____

____ mg

139. Ritalin 15 mg/M²/dose is recommended. A child who weighs 22 lb and is average in height for weight would receive how much?

BSA ____

____ mg

140. Phenobarbital 180 mg/M²/24 hr given every eight hours is recommended. How much should a child whose BSA = 0.29 receive? _____ mg

141. For a child less than five years of age, the recommended dose of Rifampin is 10–20 mg/kg/day. What is an acceptable range for a child weighing 24 lb? _____ mg

142. The recommended dose of Secobarbital is 3–5 mg/kg. A child weighing 16 kg might receive how much? _____ mg

143. Tetracyline 25–50 mg/kg/day given in four doses is recommended. What is an acceptable range for a child weighing 62 lb? _____ mg

144. Kanamycin 15 mg/kg/day given every 12 hours is recommended. Calculate a safe dose for a child weighing 18 lb. _____ mg

145. Phenobarbital 6 mg/kg/24 hr divided into three doses is recommended. How much would a child weighing 17 lb receive per dose? _____ mg

146. Cytoxan 2–3 mg/kg/24 hr is recommended. A child who weighs 32 lb would receive how much? _____ mg

147. Demerol 6 mg/kg/24 hr divided into six doses is recommended. A child weighing 16 kg should receive _____ mg per dose.

148. A drug is to be given at 20 ml/hr. If the drug is available as 800 mg/500 ml of fluid and the patient weighs 220 lb, how many mcg/kg/min is the patient receiving? _____ mcg/kg/min

149. Give Brevibloc at a rate of 250 mcg/kg/min. If the patient weighs 60 kg, how many mcg will be administered per minute?

_____ mcg/min

150. Aminophylline 30 mg/hr is ordered. The drug is available as 1 g/500 ml of fluid. At what rate should the infusion set be programmed per hour?

_____ ml/hr

151. Give Lidocaine 30 mcg/kg/min to a patient weighing 55 lb. The drug is mixed 120 mg in 100 ml D_5 W. How many mcg/min will be given? What will the infusion pump rate be?

_____ mcg/min   _____ ml/hr

152. Give Heparin 0.15 Units/kg/min from a solution mixed 5000 U in 250 ml D_5 W. The patient weighs 75 kg. How many U/min and U/hr will be given? What is the infusion pump rate?

_____ U/min   _____ U/hr   _____ ml/hr

ANSWERS

Comprehensive Exam (pp. 165–177)

1. 93.2°F	**11.** 17.3 cc	**21.** 14,500 ml, $14\frac{1}{2}$ qt
2. 47.2°C	**12.** 0.014 g	**22.** $\frac{1}{100}$ gr
3. 0.324 L	**13.** 86.36 cm	**23.** $3\frac{3}{4}$ gr, 0.25 g
4. 16,500 cc	**14.** 50.787 in	**24.** 8 gtt
5. 10,500 L	**15.** 24 ℥, 4 ʒ	**25.** 220 lb, 100,000,000 mg
6. 16,700 g	**16.** 2.2 cc	**26.** 0.12 mg
7. 3,200,000 mcg	**17.** $\frac{1}{2}$ ʒ, 1 Tbsp	**27.** $1\frac{1}{2}$ qt
8. 20 mcg	**18.** 143 lb	**28.** 3 ml
9. 0.0394 kg	**19.** $\frac{1}{2}$ pt, $8\frac{1}{3}$ ʒ	**29.** 15 ml
10. 0.000164 kl	**20.** $\frac{1}{6000}$ gr	

30. 64 ml

31. 1 gal

32. 3 mg

33. 500 mg, 0.5 g

34. 480 ml

35. 1000 ml

36. $\frac{3}{4}$ glass

37. 0.5 ml

38. 10 ml or 12.5 ml

39. 12 mg, 0.012 g

40. 0.5 mg

41. 900 ml

42. 6000 ml

43. 1 ml

44. 300 ml

45. 1 gal

46. 150 ml or 160 ml

47. 0.36 g, 360 mg

48. 8 tsp

49. 3 qt

50. 200 mg

51. 6 ml

52. 4 tab

53. 10 ml

54. 10 ml

55. 2 cap

56. $\frac{1}{2}$ tab

57. 5 ml

58. $\frac{1}{2}$ tab

59. 12.5 ml

60. 1 tsp

61. $\frac{1}{2}$ tab

62. 2 cap

63. 4 ml

64. 0.7 ml

65. 1.25 ml

66. 5 tab

67. 30 ml

68. 2 cap

69. 2 ml

70. 2 ml

71. 2.5 ml

72. 1.5 ml

73. 2.5 ml

74. 2 ml

75. 7.5 ml

76. 0.4 ml

77. 2 ml

78. 0.5 ml

79. 4 ml

80. 3 ml

81. 5 ml

82. 1 ml

83. 2.5 ml

84. 4 m_x

85. 0.8 ml

86. 0.2 ml

87. 2.5 ml

88. 5 ml

89. 20 ml

90. 1.25 ml

91. 0.5 ml

92. 3.75 ml

93. 1 ml

94. 3 ml

95. 0.4 ml

96. Dilaudid 0.75 ml
    Robinul 1 ml

97. 0.2 ml

98. 60

99. 17

100. 40

101. 20

102. 60

103. 38

104. 28

105. 36

106. 16

107. 6

108. 50

109. 75

110. 58

111. 10

112. 14

113. 42

114. 75

115. 100

116. 19

117. 14

118. 35

119. 31

120. 10

121. 21

122. 83

123. 0.02 mg

124. 0.065 g

125. $\frac{1}{50}$ gr

126. 74.4 mg

127. 65 mg

128. $\frac{1}{5000}$ gr

129. 88,200 U

130. 6 mEq

131. BSA 0.52
0.06 mg

132. BSA 0.38
8.78 mg

133. BSA 0.62
216,000 U

134. 5.2 mg

135. BSA 0.28
40 mg

136. BSA 0.8
69.36 mg

137. BSA 0.58
8.7 mg

138. BSA 1.46
8.76 mg

139. BSA 0.47
7 mg

140. 52.2 mg

141. 109–218 mg

142. 48–80 mg

143. 704.5–1409
mg/day
176–352 mg/dose

144. 61.35 mg

145. 15.46 mg

146. 29–43.5 mg

147. 16 mg

148. 5.33
mcg/kg/min

149. 15,000 mcg/min

150. 15 ml/hr

151. 750 mcg/min
38 ml/hr

152. 11.25 U/min
675 U/hr
34 ml/hr

Index